Ethics for Global Mental Health

Ethics for Global Mental Health examines the limitations of current normative approaches to global mental health (GMH) work and argues for a values-based framework that prioritizes accountability and contextual relevance of humanitarian and profession-specific values. It cautions against using aspirational ideals as operational guidance. Chapters are organized around challenges arising in humanitarian research, disaster relief, post-conflict recovery, fieldwork, and refugee resettlement and are designed to equip readers with strategies for resolving professional dilemmas and negotiating conflicting priorities. Also included is a sample training curriculum as well as case studies and exercises that help professionals address countertransference and burnout, and recognize ethically questionable practices such as trauma tourism, rescuer fantasy, or savior complex.

Elena Cherepanov, PhD, is a professor at Cambridge College where she founded one of the first certificate programs in trauma studies in the United States. She is also the behavioral health lead for refugee-integrated care at Lynn Community Health Center in Massachusetts. Dr. Cherepanov received a Carol Hacker Award for her excellence in trauma work and has worked across the globe with multiple humanitarian organizations. She is the author of over 50 papers and books translated into different languages.

Ethics for Global Mental Health

From Good Intentions to Humanitarian Accountability

Elena Cherepanov

Routledge
Taylor & Francis Group
NEW YORK AND LONDON

First published 2019
by Routledge
711 Third Avenue, New York, NY 10017

and by Routledge
2 Park Square, Milton Park, Abingdon, Oxon, OX14 4RN

Routledge is an imprint of the Taylor & Francis Group, an informa business

Library of Congress Cataloging-in-Publication Data
Names: Cherepanov, Elena, author.
Title: Ethics for global mental health : from good intentions to
humanitarian accountability / Elena Cherepanov.
Description: New York : Routledge, 2019. |
Includes bibliographical references and index.
Identifiers: LCCN 2018010281 | ISBN 9780815386209 (hbk : alk. paper) |
ISBN 9780815386223 (pbk : alk. paper) | ISBN 9781351175746 (ebk)
Subjects: LCSH: Psychiatric ethics. | Mental health services–Moral and ethical aspects.
Classification: LCC RC455.2.E8 C44 2019 | DDC 174.2/9689–dc23
LC record available at https://lccn.loc.gov/2018010281

ISBN: 978-0-815-38620-9 (hbk)
ISBN: 978-0-815-38622-3 (pbk)
ISBN: 978-1-351-17574-6 (ebk)

Typeset in Minion
by Out of House Publishing

With gratitude to my parents, Yulia and Michael Ianotovsky, for their never-ending patience, support, and encouragement.

With love to my son Peter whose moving out made this book possible.

With appreciation to the Red to Black Editing Company, my editors who always knew what I meant when I thought I spoke English.

Contents

List of Figures x
List of Tables xi
Abbreviations and Acronyms xii
Preface xv

Introduction and Overview 1

1 **Global Mental Health in a Changing World** 10
1.1 Defining Global Mental Health: "Global" and "Mental" and "Health." Oh My! 10
1.2 History of Global Mental Health: Quest for Consistency and Standards 14
1.3 Controversies and the Grand Challenges 22

2 **Contemporary Humanitarianism** 27
2.1 Understanding Contemporary Humanitarianism and its Challenges 27
2.2 History of Humanitarian Values 28
2.3 Emerging Trends in Humanitarian Action: Professionalization and Accountability 31

3 **Humanitarian Ethics** 37
3.1 Humanitarian Charter: Minimum Standards for Humanitarian Response 37
3.2 The NGO Code of Conduct 40
3.3 Ethics of Global Mental Health 42
3.4 Developing an Ethical Framework 45

4 Professional and Personal Challenges in Humanitarian Work 49
4.1 Humanitarian Crisis, Complex Emergency, and Post-Crisis Recovery 49
4.2 Role of Global Mental Health Professionals in Settings with Complex Needs: IASC and CBPR Models 52
4.3 External, Professional, and Personal Challenges 57
4.4 Exercise: Check Your Knowledge 58

5 Managing Ethical Challenges in Global Mental Health 60
5.1 Humanitarian Research. Children as Research Subjects 60
5.2 Trauma Work: Professional and Personal Boundaries 70
5.3 Disaster Mental Health: "Hurry Up and Wait" 71
5.4 Ethical Challenges in Post-Conflict Settings: What to Do with the Fish? 72
5.5 Fieldwork 76
5.6 Case Study Exercise: Navigating Ethical Dilemmas in Fieldwork 81

6 Aspirational Guidance: Principles of Humanitarian Assistance 83
6.1 Fundamental Principles of Humanitarian Assistance 83
6.2 Humanitarian Principles as Aspirational Guidance: A Moral Compass 84
6.3 Humanitarian Accountability or "Nothing About Us Without Us" 88
6.4 Exercise: Using an Aspirational Framework for Decision-Making 91

7 Operational Guidance: IASC Guidelines 94
7.1 IASC Core Principles: Consistency and Coordination 94
7.2 The Role of Ethics in Operations 95
7.3 Exercise: Using Operational Guidance for Designing Ethical Interventions 101

8 Ethical Dilemmas: Damned If You Do and Damned If You Don't 103
8.1 Ethical Dilemmas in Global Mental Health 103
8.2 Reconciling Multidisciplinary Agendas: Engaging a Higher Level of Values 104
8.3 Managing Professional Dilemmas: Establishing Accountability 106
8.4 Negotiating Moral Conundrums: A Heuristic Approach 110
8.5 Exercise: Unsolvable Conundrums—What Would You Do? 113

9 Ethically Questionable Practices 115
9.1 Countertransference: A Threat to Professional and Personal Boundaries 115
9.2 Cognitive Biases, Power Differential, and Privileges 118
9.3 Ethically Questionable Practices and Medication Misuse 119

10 Safety Imperative and Self-Care 128
10.1 Mental Health Impact of Humanitarian Work 128
10.2 A Safety Imperative 129
10.3 "We Must Not Multiply Victims" 131
10.4 Recognizing Burnout 132
10.5 Burnout Prevention and Reversal 135
10.6 Reentry or "The Other Life" 135
10.7 Exercises: Preparing for Reentry 138

11 Values-Based Ethical Framework and Core Competencies in Global Mental Health 139
11.1 Methodology of Ethical Framework 139
11.2 Values-Based Ethics: Strategies for Decision-Making 140
11.3 Professional Competencies of an Ethical Global Mental Health Specialist 141

12 Ethical Considerations for Refugee Mental Health Providers in the United States 146
12.1 Refugee Mental Health: Current Developments and Professional Challenges 147
12.2 Values and Competencies of an Ethical Refugee Mental Health Provider 150
12.3 Cognitive Biases and Self-Care 152
12.4 Case Studies: Negotiating Ethical Dilemmas 155

13 Conclusion and Future Directions 161
13.1 Summary 161
13.2 Future Directions 164
13.3 Conclusion 165

Appendix 1: Ethics for Global Mental Health: Training Curriculum 6–8 Hours 167
Appendix 2: Boston Globe *Letter* 172
References 174
Index 189

Figures

1.1	"The World Would Be a Better Place If …"	25
2.1	Accountability	33
3.1	Aid Unintended Effects	39
3.2	Life with Dignity	40
3.3	The System of Values Governing Global Mental Health	46
3.4	Interplay Between Multidisciplinary and Professional Values in Global Mental Health	47
4.1	Classification of Humanitarian Emergencies	50
4.2	IASC Intervention Pyramid for Mental Health and Psychosocial Supports in Emergencies	53
5.1	"Give Man a Fish …"	73
7.1	"Actually, I Was Hoping for a More Inspiring Mission Statement"	98
8.1	Engagement of Humanitarian Values to Reconcile the Conflicting Multidisciplinary Agenda	106
8.2	Accountability in Professional Dilemmas	109
8.3	Reasoning Moral Dilemmas	112
9.1	"Barbie Savior"	123
9.2	How to Communicate with the World: A Social Media Guide for Volunteers and Travelers	125
10.1	10 Ways to Be Happier Today	135

Tables

1.1	Defining Global Mental Health	12
1.2	5Rs Model: Operational Modalities in Global Mental Health	13
1.3	History of Global Mental Health	21
2.1	Abbreviated History of Humanitarian Values	32
3.1	Professional Code of Ethics (Normative Ethics) and the Ethics of GMH (Values-Based Framework)	44
5.1	Ethical Challenges in Humanitarian and Global Mental Health Research	63
5.2	An MSF Ethical Framework for Humanitarian Innovations	78
9.1	The Belief System of the White Savior Industrial Complex	117
9.2	Cognitive Biases in Global Mental Health	120
10.1	Factors Undermining the Safety Imperative	131
10.2	Burnout: Indicators and Contributing Causes	134
10.3	Strategies for Burnout Prevention and Reversal	136
10.4	Return from Mission: Normal Versus Complicated Reentry	137
11.1	Professional Competencies of an Ethical Global Mental Health Specialist	144
12.1	Current Developments in Refugee Mental Health	148
12.2	Challenges in Mental Health Work with Refugees	149
12.3	Aspirational Values in Refugee Mental Health	150
12.4	Operational Guidelines in Refugee Mental Health	151

Abbreviations and Acronyms

APA	American Psychological Association
ATSS	Association of Traumatic Stress Specialists
CBPR	community-based psychological recovery in complex emergency model
CCAPS	climate change and African political stability
CE	complex emergency
GBV	gender-based violence
GMH	global mental health
HAP	humanitarian accountability partnership
IASC	inter-agency standing committee
IFRC	International Federation of the Red Cross
IPV	intimate partner violence
LLMIC	low- and lower-middle-income countries
M&E	monitoring and evaluation
MGMH	Movement for Global Mental Health
MH	mental health
mhGAP	Mental Health Global Action Plan
MHPSS	mental health and psychosocial supports
MSF	Médicins Sans Frontières
NGO	non-governmental organization
NIMBY	"Not in my backyard!"
NIMH	National Institute of Mental Health
OCHA	Office for the Coordination of Humanitarian Affairs

RMH	refugee mental health
SAMHSA	Substance Abuse and Mental Health Services Administration
SDGs	sustainable development goals
SDH	social determinants of heath
TB	tuberculosis
UN	United Nations
UNHCR	United Nations High Commission for Refugees
WHO	World Health Organization
WHS	World Humanitarian Summit
WTF	World Trauma Foundation

Preface

This book is a labor of love dedicated to the humanitarians, whose tireless nomadic souls are always and forever my inspiration

I have come to recognize humanitarians by their eyes. In many ways, they are like everyone else. They pursue education and careers, fall in and out of love, pay mortgages, get frustrated with bosses, and enjoy a glass (or three) of wine with friends. Yet, there is something intrinsically different about them. Like in Ray Bradbury's Martians, their eyes both reflect the harsh winds of faraway lands we will never see and hide a kind of knowledge that strips away pretense and starkly reveals the true value of things.

Coming back from field assignment has always been the hardest part. In the field, the "real life" back at home gradually and insidiously recedes into the distance. Daily work routines and even small pleasures slip into the empty spots in their concept of "normal." One night, on the brink of falling asleep, they realize with a terrified skip of their hearts that they have not thought about "home" for an entire day. Home has become a detached and abstract concept.

Once they recognize this symptom, they work hard at persuading themselves that of course they do care about home … they just cannot admit to themselves that they no longer do. Nostalgia requires leisure and privacy, something fieldwork lacks in abundance.

"Here" and "there" trade places in a field life with alarming ease. Each part of their existence become a world of its own. What gives the purpose and value to their lives in one world seem pointless and worthless in the other. Once in a while, a seismic cataclysm cracks open the fault lines in their reality and the blazingly bright memory lane brings them back home with the mercilessness sharp realization that they have chosen a world that doesn't care about them over being with those who do need, love, and worry about them. They shelter themselves against this brutal truth, using crushing workloads, numbing routines, or partying like there's no tomorrow.

As the time for returning home approaches, counting hours becomes an obsession. They are still enjoying the bittersweet comfort of inside jokes with fellow expatriates but the mind already wonders away and fantasizes about what will be the first thing they do or eat. And only much later they realize that the food they dreamed about does not taste as good as they imagined, friends are busy doing other things, colleagues have advanced in their careers, and family begin to get glassy-eyed when they mention "the field."

The airplane, like an aluminum time capsule, connects time and space and gently transition them into a world that they call home. At the terminal, they feel awkward in the colorful crowd and recognize other aid workers by their ragged backpacks, worn hiking shows, and dazed look. You probably spot them sitting in the corner alone or comfortably sleeping in the most uncomfortable place. They seems to avoid casual conversations and have low tolerance for chitchat.

When at home, they find that their family is overjoyed and relieved to see them. They are genuinely trying to spend more quality time with family and friends, which quickly turns into exhausting duty because of the emotional disconnect. They discover that nothing that they journaled in the field speaks to their heart. They don't even know why they wrote it in the first place. Suddenly, they realize that they are simply strangers in a strange land once more, and they must begin again to learn the customs of the place.

And then they return to work, where they fake excitement about the new color of walls or sales numbers. It is not only difficult to empathize with co-workers about the limited gluten-free vegan meal selection at the hospital cafeteria, but also they genuinely wonder why are they expected to treat people who are not dying. Lucky are those who don't lose their job over the brutal honesty when telling bosses that they can no longer ignore the social injustice in the work place.

All this weighs so heavy that going to the next mission immediately seems like an easy way out.

If they chose to stay, eventually life starts feeling normal, and they stop telling the "field stories" after realizing that no one cares, and they no longer freak out seeing food thrown away.

What is left? Becoming restless when hearing the news that somewhere war broke out, and sick to the stomach when learning of yet another fallen aid worker. There also is a warmth of comradeship and saying "be safe" instead of goodbye.[1]

This book is very important for me. It organizes my observations, thoughts, and accumulated years of experience that in the process of writing somehow came together like pieces of a puzzle.

As I looked back, many things suddenly become clear. I have always enjoyed imagining what my life would be like if I had lived somewhere else; what I would do if life got really tough. Growing up in the former Soviet Union, my fantasies were fed off reading about travel and adventures in faraway lands. I never imagined being able to freely travel internationally and that my curiosity would take me around the world.

My interest in trauma started in the 1980s when we, enthusiastic psychology students in Moscow, led heated discussions about how psychology could save the world. There, I first heard about psychologists who volunteered to support people affected by wars or disasters. I was impressed by one of them who told a story about how he joined the resistance during one ethnic conflict. He ended up fighting and was even lightly wounded. This image of "the glorious psychologist with a gun who is ready to fight for his clients" was so powerfully imprinted in my soul that only many years later did it started losing its appeal.

I don't know the real reason why I am drawn to this work. The desire to help others is definitely not it. The global work does satisfy my professional curiosity, give my work meaning, and make me feel needed. But there is something else: as one of my colleagues said, "it almost feels that we have no choice."

First was Spitak, the devastating earthquake in Armenia in December of 1988 when almost 50,000 people were killed after poorly built houses imploded, burying entire schools. There I saw how communities can come together in the wake of devastation. The discipline of disaster mental health was making its first steps and we were equipped with good intentions, Rogerian active listening skills, and some expressive art therapy ideas. We were learning as we went, and I am still ashamed of how unprepared we were while pretending that we knew what we were doing. There I first noticed that a disaster invokes not only the best but also the worst in people. There were bizarre volunteers "flocking in" who called themselves professionals but had no credentials, expertise, or affiliations; psychologists were using experimental methods and psychiatrists were giving away medication like candy without even talking to survivors. I also saw how quickly compassion turned into victim-blaming. They were accused of "playing victim" so they could get more help, or of "not appreciating the aid." After the initial shock, I became fascinated with recognizing the same attitudes in different settings, countries, and cultures. That was the first time I realized that humanitarian relief requires professionalism, special expertise, and skills.

In 1989–1993, I trained local psychologists, teachers, and nurses after the Chernobyl nuclear power plant disaster. They lived and worked in the areas exposed to radiation and they taught me that hope for the future in seemingly hopeless situations can come from past survivorship ("We survived the war!") and a "one day at a time" attitude. In Chernobyl, I saw the devastating impact of inadequate information about the real scale of a disaster igniting rumors, misinformation, and distrust in official sources. When evacuated, the survivors faced stigmatization and isolation similar to the survivors after the Hiroshima and

Nagasaki bombings, and later after the Fukushima nuclear disaster, as a colleague from Japan shared with me in private conversation.

And then was the Chechen war in 1996, where I came to understand that in war, casualties come from both sides. There I saw the Russian military, the 18-year-old boys who had just left their warm and loving families, after they had killed so as not to get killed themselves. I also came to realize the unforgiving power of traditional culture when Chechen teenagers—who never cry and in the absence of the men take full responsibility for the whole family—asked about their future plans would tell me that the plan was to graduate school and avenge the death of their parents. I remember the horrifying realization that ethnic conflicts never end, they just become dormant, and that psychologists can play the role in breaking this never-ending cycle.

While working in the camps with Kosovo refugees, I was able to observe the "magic" of humanitarian medicine, as the humanitarian anthropologist Sharon Abramowitz (2015, p. 139) called the humanitarian medical NGOs' capacity to construct an effective institutional apparatus that could sustain the delivery of basic and complex health services, surgical care, and public health intervention in an environment of extreme flux. I was fascinated by the capacity of humanitarian relief when almost overnight the agencies erected a tent city for tens of thousands of refugees, which had infrastructure, security, schools, and health care facilities, where each NGO knew their role and worked collaboratively and complementarily. There I learned about the dual function of the refugee camps to meet basic needs for displaced people and also to provide basic protection against those who may not want to have refugees "in their backyards." On a personal level, working with Kosovo refugees powerfully reminded me about the fragility of everything that I wanted to believe were the primary and indestructible elements of humanity: human connection, community and neighborhood, family ties, love, and friendship. When civil war breaks out, all this becomes a threat and burden that diminishes chances for survivorship. When hearing stories about how neighbors, childhood friends, and family members turned against each other, I had a flashback to Stalin's repressions in the 1930s, when many were murdered after their friends, coworkers, or even family members turned them over to KGB or denounced them as the enemies of the people.

Training the trauma responders in the Ukraine reinforced my belief that our helping profession helps us to remain sane when the world around us is shattered into pieces, and respond to human suffering regardless of the political affiliation.

My work in Liberia taught me that provision of aid can be an extremely delicate task that needs to be well planned to protect the dignity of desperate people and to prevent violent competition for resources. There I had the privilege to meet Dr. Janice Cooper, who felt that, as a Liberian, she had an obligation to put in place something solid and to be accountable for the dollars that were invested. I learned from her about the importance of staying the course, fighting for what you believe, striving for excellence, and not setting a different standard for Africa or for LMICs.

My global mental health (GMH) work with vulnerable people has made me proud of my profession and helped me to realize the true scale of the damage that can be done by unregulated and unethical practices. These concerns became the primary reason for writing this book.

This book is not intended for those who show intentional and callous disregard for life, safety, and the well-being of others, but rather for those globally minded specialists and students who are inspired to join the humanitarian cause. In humanitarian work, nothing is what it seems, nothing works as intended, and simple solutions never work—even the best intentions can cause harm if they are not supported by professionalism. When facing the abyss of human suffering, deciding what is right and what is wrong can be a daunting task, and then ethics provide guidance and support with difficult moral dilemmas.

I do not promise to solve all the problems or offer peace of mind to readers. Instead, I aim to foster dialog, explore gray areas, and raise questions. In the process of developing the model for an ethical framework, this book touches upon dynamic and sensitive issues of professional and international affairs. In some cases, the situations and the opinions described here will have already changed by the time of its publication because of new information or data that has become available; in other cases, new trends and understandings should emerge. For understandable reasons, I will refrain from criticizing specific organizations, individuals, and governments, instead offering generic case studies. The hypothetical scenarios for exercises are loosely based on real-life cases that have been altered to avoid references to identifiable providers, regions, or agencies.

My hope is that this book helps those interested in GMH to realize that having "good intentions" is not enough—this work requires rigorous training and professional competencies.

Note

1 I want to thank Cait Reynolds who helped me to narrate this piece.

Introduction and Overview

Introduction

GMH professionals respond to ever-increasing humanitarian needs and provide mental health (MH) supports and advocacy to populations affected by wars, armed conflicts, disasters, famines, or severe poverty. They conduct research, advise on MH policies, help to build local capacity, support aid workers, and train local specialists. Some of them work independently, but most are employed by nongovernmental organizations (NGOs) or private charitable foundations.

GMH branched out as a professional specialization at the end of the 1980s, when globally minded MH professionals became acutely aware of the scale of emergencies and suffering around the world and felt that they could and should help in their professional capacity. They also were interested to learn about the world through how people from different cultures cope with life adversities.

The international experience broadened the horizons of the profession, demonstrated the power of human resilience, and revived interest in cultural diversity. It also demonstrated that serving the most vulnerable populations comes with responsibility and requires specialized professional competencies. The global perspective deepened our understanding of the role of MH work and allowed an honest and uncompromised evaluation of its core assumptions, achievements, and shortfalls. The followed paradigmatic shift challenged the self-centered and at times naïve convictions about the universality and transferability of professional skills to different cultures and contexts. It also revealed limitations of the biomedical model of MH, with its reduction of the complex reality of trauma and normal human responses to life adversities to a set of pathological symptoms.

A literature review and analysis of the professional challenges, endowed with my own experience, were used to examine different dimensions of GMH work, including the sometimes contradictory views on its professional agenda and values. By virtue of being at the crossroads of the globalization of humanitarianism, the mission of GMH has many times been called into question over its covert and overt agendas. Ironically, the arising controversies and harsh critique of GMH increased its public visibility, facilitated its professional self-determination, and made it a testing ground for different concepts and best practices. As a result of these efforts, the GMH that started as voluntaristic and fragmented efforts has emerged in a short period of time on the global stage as a vital humanitarian actor without which we cannot imagine the contemporary multidisciplinary humanitarianism.

In this role, GMH joined a number of global initiatives prioritizing accountability and quality assurance (Sphere, 2004), and this book has been envisioned as part of this agenda. In humanitarian work where the effectiveness of the relief efforts by and large depends on the consistency and quality of collaborations, ethical guidance plays an essential role in ensuring accountability, and flagging unethical practices. The transgression of ethical values, on the other hand, undermines the spirit of humanitarianism, drastically affects the ability of agencies to respond to survivors' needs, and puts aid workers and the people they serve at risk.

Global work takes MH professionals out of their comfort zones and forces them to reexamine everything they thought they knew about the profession, the world, and themselves. In their work they often encounter unique moral and unprecedented professional dilemmas. Their ethics offer professional grounding, set expectations, and establish a frame of reference for practice and professional interactions that are consistent with humanitarian values and strengthen the image of the humanitarian profession.

Ethicists who studied ethical challenges in humanitarian research, disaster relief, traumatology, fieldwork, and refugee MH pointed out the limitations of normative professional standards and highlighted the need for a broader frame of reference. In contrast to reliance on predetermined norms, standards, and protocols, a values-based framework allows for establishing the contextual relevance of ethical imperatives and indicates which to prioritize when approaching a complex problem. The flexibility and situational congruency of this approach comes at a price: its adoption places more responsibility on the provider in the decision-making process and elevates the roles of professional judgment, professional competency, and personal integrity.

In order to provide guidance for the collaborative, complementary, and consistent humanitarian response, the values of GMH integrate those shared by other multidisciplinary humanitarian actors (universal humanitarian values) with those that are the profession-specific. While professional codes of ethics always remain at the core of any decision-making for a professional, the competencies- and values-based framework allows for making choices that are consistent with humanitarian values, minimize harm, and assure professional accountability. Prioritizing values does not equate to prioritizing MH needs. Instead, it reflects establishing contextual relevance and a primacy of values for professional decision-making in different contexts.

The proposed values-based framework for GMH can guide navigation of moral ambiguities and intractable professional dilemmas that reflect the underlying conflict of paradigms. Within this framework, accountability, professional competencies, and self-awareness play central roles for making truly informed choices and reconciling competing agendas and paradigms. For example, when multidisciplinary agendas compete, MH professionals can contribute to securing the willingness of stakeholders to engage in the dialog about prioritizing the needs of an affected population.

Whether MH professionals serve populations impacted by humanitarian crises internationally or they provide MH services for refugees at the places of their resettlement, they encounter professional dilemmas that go beyond routine clinical practice. The humanitarian commitment introduces a "bigger picture" for our professional role and responsibility in ambiguous situations. For example, when we cannot determine which value is "more professional" or "more moral," the humanitarian principles and accountability can help decide which value is more consistent with the humanitarian ideals, leading to less harm and the greatest benefits for those being helped.

It is important to note that humanitarian principles form a living document that continuously evolves to reflect the changing understanding of modern humanitarianism and emerging themes. They serve as aspiration or a moral compass but do not provide practical solutions. The operational guidance is based on the *Guidelines on Mental Health and Psychosocial Support in Emergency Settings* developed by IASC (2007) where the role of ethics is to assure that the operational recommendations are implemented in a professional and morally responsible way.

The professional and personal challenges of humanitarian work, not surprisingly, put a heavy emotional burden on and affect the psychological well-being of GMH professionals, who often work in physically demanding and unsafe settings where they have to make quick and effective decisions under duress in situations with a high degree of moral ambiguity. The Antares Foundation (Young, 2015) found that 79 percent of the 754 respondents to the survey on the *Guardian* Global Development Professional Network reported that they had experienced MH issues related to their fieldwork. This research points out the psychological and MH needs of aid workers and positions safety, self-care, and burnout prevention as core professional competencies.

This book recognizes ethical challenges and intends to equip providers with practical strategies for managing them and negotiating the conflicts of multidisciplinary, professional, and moral values. It offers tools for increasing self-awareness and self-care, and encourages the understanding of safety as professional imperatives. The case studies at the end of chapters illustrate these dilemmas, allow practicing problem-solving strategies, and can be used as training or supervisory tools. This book:

- examines the role of GMH in a changing world, defines its scope of services, and identifies its main challenges;
- explores historical milestones, the current state, and future directions for GMH;
- determines the need and establishes a values-based ethical framework for GMH work that includes aspirational values shared by the multidisciplinary actors and profession-specific operational values;

- inspects ethical challenges, conflicts of multidisciplinary agendas, professional dilemmas, and moral conundrums in different aspects of GMH work, and offers strategies for decision-making;
- recognizes the role of self-awareness in forestalling ethically questionable practices;
- affirms the safety imperative and self-care as ethical requirements and core professional competencies;
- offers case examples to practice reasoning through the dilemmas;
- provides a sample of the curriculum for training the ethics of GMH.

Overview

Chapter 1 defines GMH and examines its history, mission, and current trends. It reviews different approaches to conceptualizing GMH and proposes its understanding as *an area of study and practice that aims to support psychological recovery and to improve psychological well-being in populations affected by international humanitarian crises*—whereas according to mhGAP (2008), MH is understood as a state of well-being in which every individual realizes his or her own potential, can cope with the normal stresses of life, can work productively and fruitfully, and is able to make a contribution to her or his community.

Although MH interventions have been implemented since the 1980s, this is the first time when GMH is clearly defined as a professional specialization with a dual MH and humanitarian professional identity. It is suggested that the uniqueness of its scope of services in GMH is determined by its humanitarian context, the complex emergency setting, the complex needs of its target populations, and the modalities of its interventions (5Rs model: Relief, Response, Recovery, Reinforcement, and Retention).

The historical perspective of GMH helps to better understand how it has come to be what it is now. Although humanitarian spirit has always drawn people to help those who are in greater need, the professional self-determination of GMH can be traced to three major developments: (a) the inclusion of a PTSD diagnosis in the *Diagnostic and Statistical Manual of Mental Disorders* (DSM-III) in 1980, (b) the growing interest in multicultural diversity, and (c) the globalization of humanitarianism.

The GMH that initially started as voluntaristic and fragmented efforts based on good intentions moved to implementing empirically developed psychosocial and primary care integrated models that became the gold standards of GMH practice. The growth and diversification of the programs that followed highlighted the need for consistency, standards, and regulations, leading GMH to join global humanitarian initiatives focusing on increasing professionalization and accountability in humanitarian action. As part of this global agenda, the Grand Challenges project was set to develop a roadmap to identify and address the main challenges in GMH.

By being in the center of the controversies pertaining to the globalization of the humanitarian movement and proliferation of Western concepts of MH, GMH opened itself to transformative global processes and the associated "war of paradigms" that underscored the importance of establishing an ethical framework to ensure the standards and integrity of practice.

Chapter 2 reflects upon contemporary humanitarianism—the historical evolution of its values, current controversies, and emerging themes. While the significance of humanitarian ideals is never in question, the principles and values continue to develop along with the increasing understanding of the complexity of humanitarian action—and also of its limitations. The adoption of humanitarian values was initially driven by the need to establish a common values-based framework for humanitarian action and to make actors agree on basic principles. The globalization and industrialization of humanitarianism put up front the professionalization and humanitarian accountability, which was understood as responsibility toward both stakeholders and the use of power and resources. The focus on accountability has led service providers to question whether they were the ones who were supposed to decide about what the population needs. The accountability-centered approach encourages engaging stakeholders and eliciting their feedback at every step of decision-making about humanitarian interventions and partnering with them in the process of implementing the interventions, or "nothing about us without us!"

Chapter 3 talks about the role of the Sphere Project in establishing consistency and coordination among humanitarian actors with different missions and agendas. The Sphere Project pioneered minimum standards for the humanitarian charter and emergency response. The humanitarian charter captures both the ethical and legal foundations of humanitarian action and is defined as an expression of the current consensus in the humanitarian community (Sphere, 2004). In an effort to move the human rights agenda forward and establish protection for beneficiaries, the prominent NGOs adopted the Code of Conduct that sets up consistent conduct expectations for humanitarian workers—because a tarnished image increases risks for humanitarians and less lifesaving aid.

It is proposed that the ethical framework for GMH be defined as the system of professional and multidisciplinary values, competencies, and standards that provide guidance and a frame of reference for reasoning the complex professional and moral dilemmas arising within the humanitarian context.

Ethicists demonstrated the limitations of normative ethics in the unprecedented and morally ambiguous situations that GMH providers encounter in abundance. Values-based ethics, on the contrary, enable establishing contextual relevance of ethical imperatives and rely on professional competency in determining which one to follow.

The multidisciplinary and cross-sectional values adopted by the humanitarian community are built upon universal human rights and the humanitarian principles that are the humanitarian imperative, accountability, impartiality, neutrality, non-proselytism, and not taking advantage of aid recipients' vulnerabilities

(IFRC, 1965; Sphere, 2004). Whereas humanitarian values represent aspirational ideals, IASC guidelines (2007) provide operational guidance; the professional codes are binding, and safety and self-care are imperative for any humanitarian affiliate regardless of the professional identity.

Chapter 4 defines the external, personal, and professional challenges the GMH providers face when working in complex emergencies. A "complex emergency" (CE) is characterized by extensive violence and loss of life, massive displacements of people, widespread damage to societies and economies, the need for large-scale, multifaceted humanitarian assistance, and the hindrance or prevention of humanitarian assistance by political and military constraints (WHO, 2002). To address the complex needs of affected populations and ensure implementation of coordinated MH agenda, IASC issued the guidelines for MH and psychosocial supports in emergencies (IASC, 2007), which designate the roles for providers within a multi-layered and complementary system of MH interventions. This needs-based model serves as operational guidance for determining the best course of action when the choice of interventions is limited by politics, funding, resources, or compromised referral systems.

Chapter 5 uses literature reviews and field reports to identify ethical challenges in different facets of GMH work: humanitarian research, trauma work, disaster response, post-conflict settings, and fieldwork. Ethical challenges and their management are discussed in relation to the limitations of the existing normative frameworks and the need for broadening the ethical paradigm to make it relevant to GMH work.

The IASC (2014), which declared *humanitarian research* a priority component of GMH, identified the main ethical challenges and suggested strategies for addressing them in the areas of validity, confidentiality, potential for inflicting emotional distress, informed consent, and the researcher's responsibility. It is suggested that the participatory model of the research can mitigate some of these challenges. According to Cherepanov (2017b), use of children as research subjects calls for an additional layer of protection due to children's vulnerability and dependence on adults.

Trauma work is a big part of the GMH mandate. Williams (2012) believed that exposure to severe trauma and suffering triggers countertransference that erodes professional and personal boundaries and is a main cause of problematic judgments and burnout in traumatologists. She suggested that self-care is not only a professional competency, but also an ethical requirement for traumatologists.

The ethical challenges in *disaster management* relate to crisis response and the emergency mode of the interventions, which place almost sole responsibility for risk management and harm reduction on the responder who must balance multiple priorities while maintaining the integrity of professional interventions, such as confidentiality. Jenson (1997) argued that, in a disaster, the traditional tools of "objective" logic, rationality, and consistency may not be adequate, and the disaster management should be primarily governed by humanitarian values.

When participating in recovery, peacemaking, or capacity building in a *post-conflict setting*, GMH providers must be able to justify that interventions are conducted for the sole benefit of the affected region and not to advance political, social, or professional agendas. This can be accomplished through strengthening accountability, which emphasizes the importance of engaging beneficiaries in decisions about their needs and goals.

Many ethical challenges encountered in fieldwork revolve around the professional and moral dilemmas with few good solutions that arise when multidisciplinary actors strive to meet the complex or competing needs of the beneficiaries.

Chapter 6 examines the aspirational role of the humanitarian principles that are shared by humanitarian actors and stresses that the aspirational values serve as a moral compass and do not provide prescriptions for operations. In their work, GMH providers will likely face dilemmas where any decision comes with a serious cost. In the context of uncertainty and conflicting values, the humanitarian principles provide a meta-level reference and offer strategic guidance for such decision-making. However, confusing ideals with operational guidance may lead to problematic outcomes, like "humanitarian military intervention" where humanitarian ideals are used to justify military interventions.

Chapter 7 analyzes the operational guidance offered by the *IASC Guidelines on Mental Health and Psychosocial Support in Emergency Settings* (IASC, 2007) and outlines the role of ethics in their implementation. Operational guidance establishes consistency in complementary interventions—or refers to "what to do"—while ethics refer to "how to do it right" as well as "what not to do." The case studies provide opportunity to practice using the operational and ethical guidelines to assure that GMH projects are designed and implemented in an ethical manner.

Chapter 8 investigates the competing multidisciplinary agendas, professional dilemmas, and moral conundrums in GMH and offers strategies for their navigation. It is proposed that these dilemmas are approached as a false opposition or the conflict of underlying paradigms that can be negotiated by establishing the contextual relevance of the meta values.

In this way, engaging humanitarian principles as higher-level values helps to negotiate the *competing multidisciplinary agenda*, like having to choose between prioritizing education or health care. In an ideal world, these agendas should not compete and should be complementary, but resources are almost always limited. It is possible, for instance, to consider prioritizing the allocation of resources based on what is more pertinent to the humanitarian principles based on the situational demands that are going to be different during the health crisis or post-conflict recovery.

When resolving *professional dilemmas*, like having to choose between an intervention that benefits an individual or one that benefits the community, exerting accountability as a point of reference helps with establishing the primacy of the value in relation to the professional role and the current commitment. This means that this decision may be different depending on the professional role of a provider (i.e. a public health provider or a clinician) at a given time and place, the agency's mission, resources, funding, and the demands of the situation. This dilemma proved to be extremely contentious during the recent Ebola outbreak in West Africa when the providers had to make a decision about quarantining a suspected case.

Reasoning *moral conundrums* calls for a heuristic approach where different levels of problem solving are recognized—which can be emotional, moral, rational, or professional—and thus helps the actor make an informed decision about the choice most appropriate for the situation.

Chapter 9 demonstrates the detrimental impact of countertransference, biases, and prejudices on professional judgment, boundaries, quality of interactions, and the integrity of care. The resultant emotional over-engagement affects the providers' MH leading to burnout. Training, supervision, and peer support aid in recognizing and managing the countertransference and gaining awareness about the power differential. Going further, the chapter describes common ethically questionable practices such as trauma tourism, rescuer fantasy, savior complex, or lacking a "sense of stage." It also brings up issues concerning potential misuse of medications.

Chapter 10 examines the impact of GMH work on the providers' psychological well-being and the role of ethics in ensuring safety and self-care. It makes the point that humanitarian work carries significant risks and exposes providers to mass suffering and mortality, which may create a perception that life has no value, resulting in neglecting self-care and/or taking unnecessary risks. In humanitarian work, the safety imperative or the absolute priority of safety refers to security and information technologies, environmental concerns, and the fundamental premise of how we assess the risks and prioritize safety. When existential despair and survivor's guilt sink in, it is very easy to lose perspective and feel that joining the victims is the only moral choice left. This is why safety and self-care are proposed to be regarded as an ethical responsibility and be included in the NGO Code of Conduct. Further on, I identify several factors that hinder compliance with the safety imperative. They are: the "dual loyalty" dilemma, "humanitarian impunity bubble," "existential despair," "a rescuer fantasy," compromised personal supports, and burnout.

Not surprisingly, the burnout rate among aid workers is extremely high (McDonald, 2015), and recognizing the indicators is the first step toward its reversal. A list of common burnout indicators is supplied along with recommendations for their reversal. Special attention is given to reentry, a time during which the returning aid workers often face difficult readjustment that may exacerbate the trauma and stresses endured during fieldwork—which, once again, emphasizes the crucial importance of self-care and peer supports.

Chapter 11 analyses how the values are organized into the values-based framework. To guide the decision-making in GMH, these values are expected to be interconnected, not contradictory, consistent with humanitarian principles, and facilitating the establishing collaborative and complementary interventions. The normative approach to ethical dilemmas may have limitations in capturing the complexity of multidisciplinary and multifactorial problems in GMH. In contrast, the values-based approach allows for balancing faithfulness to professional values with flexibility, thinking outside of the box, and situational appropriateness of decisions.

Adoption of the values-based framework elevates the role of professional competencies. This approach echoes Kohlberg's post-conventional stage of moral development (Kohlberg, 1976). Individuals who exhibit post-conventional morality view rules as useful but changeable mechanisms and apply them in contextually relevant ways while maintaining fidelity to universal moral values.

Various researchers and practitioners generally agree that an ethical GMH provider is being faithful to the humanitarian mission, having knowledge of regional history and geopolitics, possessing curiosity and respect for the different ways of life in different cultures, having trust that people are basically resilient, being able to tolerate moral ambiguities, being aware of their own limitations, and reaching out for help when needed.

Chapter 12 talks about ethical considerations for the MH professionals who service refugees resettled in the United States. This stand-alone chapter was written as a response to the refugee crisis and is organized differently from the other chapters: it presents a complete module aimed to increase ethical competencies in MH specialists or providers-in-training. While this chapter is based largely on the previously discussed findings, it focuses sharply on managing the ethical challenges that are pertinent to refugee MH work in host countries.

Globally minded providers who choose to provide MH and psychosocial support for refugees are often driven by a desire to help vulnerable populations and support the humanitarian cause. Refugees' trauma and vulnerability, anti-immigrant sentiments, and the associated biases underscore the need for high professional and ethical standards. The generic case examples help to examine dilemmas that providers have faced when working with refugees. The following discussion and recommended strategies for managing ethical challenges, along with a list of professional competencies of an ethical refugee MH provider, can be used for training and supervisory purposes.

And last, Chapter 13 summarizes the findings and outlines the directions for the future of GMH in a changing world where placing accountability at the center of the cross-sectional governance of humanitarian response allows coordinating conflicting priorities and establishing GMH as an integrated humanitarian actor. The global perspective on MH has expanded the horizon of MH practice and mainstream health care systems and reminded health care providers about their professional mission and ideals. This chapter discusses what health and MH care professionals in the United States can learn from global work to reconnect with the fundamental purpose of their profession.

CHAPTER 1

Global Mental Health in a Changing World

1.1 Defining Global Mental Health: "Global" and "Mental" and "Health." Oh My!

> What is that that mental health workers are doing, anyway?
> (E. Cherepanov, personal communication, March 4, 2015)

This question coming from a fellow aid worker was yet another reminder about the difficulties in defining GMH. How can we work on developing ethics of GMH when there is little agreement or clarity about its mission and the scope of services? This chapter examines the definitions and formulates the operational concept of GMH.

Ever since GMH appeared on the professional stage, there have been multiple attempts to capture its distinctiveness by emphasizing different aspects of this work. Historically, these different approaches to GMH were the reflection of the writers' vision of the role of MH in a changing world. Even now, when GMH has gained recognition as a vital part of humanitarian action, it still remains in the process of defining and redefining its paradigm and the scope of the services. Currently, there is a wide range of connotations associated with the term GMH, and in this book it will be used in reference to the MH work that takes place in the international humanitarian context. Next, we will examine in more detail the various working definitions of GMH that are concurrently used by the professional community.

1. The Interagency Standing Committee (IASC) describes the MH and psychosocial interventions and supports (MHPSS) as "a set of minimum multi-sectoral responses to protect and improve people's mental health and psychosocial well-being in the midst of an emergency" (IASC, 2007, p. 5). Whereas the Mental Health General Action Plan 2013–2020 defines mental health (MH), as a state of well-being in which every individual realizes his or her own potential, can cope with the normal stresses of life, can work productively and fruitfully, and is able to make a contribution to her or his community (WHO/mhGAP, 2008).

2. Patel and Prince (2010, p. 176) viewed mental illness as a trans-cultural phenomenon and approached GMH as an application of the global health principles to the domain of mental ill-health. To advance the agenda of a new field, Patel and Prince concentrated on one area of GMH work, i.e. social psychiatry, which at the time seemed to be well positioned to withstand the social and political controversies. They used Koplan, Bond, and Merson's (2009) definition of global health to specifically define GMH as the area of study, research, and practice that places a priority on improving MH and achieving equity in MH for all people worldwide. This definition does not include the psychosocial well-being that is present in the IASC definition, possibly because (this is my speculation) within medical paradigms the well-being is understood as absence of the illness. Since then, the concepts of psychological recovery, social determinants of health (SDH) and the integrated approaches (further discussed in section 1.2) broadened our understanding of the well-being as a holistic phenomenon. Patel and Prince's definition emphasized the aspirational agenda of social equity in accessing MH services, but also inadvertently added to the controversies surrounding the idea of "improving mental health," as it in some ways justified worries about pathologizing human reactions to life adversities and imposing an ethnocentric Western understanding of what "good mental health" should be (Mills, 2013; Summerfield, 2012).
3. In their book, Katz and Shoetz-Miller (2015) offered a definition that moved further away from the controversial idea of "improving mental health" toward emphasizing the role of GMH in addressing barriers to accessing MH care. Consequently, their definition stated that GMH means "the collaborative activities conducted by health, mental health, and allied mental health professionals and community and government partners that improve access to mental health care and maintenance for all people in all places" (p. 7).
4. Another way to define GMH was by its objectives. This definition is employed in the currently acting GMH action plan (WHO/mhGAP, 2010) issued by the World Health Organization (WHO), which recognizes the essential role of MH in achieving health for all people and identifies four major objectives for GMH:
   a. Strengthen effective leadership and governance for MH.
   b. Provide comprehensive, integrated, and responsive MH and social care services in the humanitarian context and community-based settings.
   c. Implement strategies for MH promotion and prevention.
   d. Strengthen information systems, evidence, and research for MH.
5. The operational definition of GMH that I use in this book underscores the humanitarian context of the work, and replaces the contentious notion of "improving mental health" with "supporting psychological recovery and promoting psychological well-being." The well-being is viewed as the contentment and the contextual congruency or doing their best under the circumstances.

> With this understanding, it is proposed that GMH is defined as an area of study and practice the goal of which is to support psychological recovery and to improve psychological well-being of populations affected by international humanitarian crises.

With this understanding, I propose that GMH is defined as *an area of study and practice the goal of which is to support psychological recovery and to improve psychological well- being of populations affected by international humanitarian crises.*

This means that the GMH as professional specialization is determined by the:

- humanitarian context;
- complex emergency setting;
- complex needs of the population it serves;
- operational modality of interventions or 5Rs model.

The context, setting and populational needs will be examined in the respective chapters, and here we will elaborate on what is the operational modality. The *operational modality* is a paraphrase of the term used by financial investment institutions (UNCC, 2011). The operational modality determines what strategies, approaches, and methods are best suited for creating an enabling environment either for short-term relief or sustainable recovery (see Table 1.1). It refers to the specific interventions in a wide variety of permutations to meet the stakeholders' needs. This also includes relevant technology and tools, information gathering and sharing, policy and institutional reforms, and capacity development. Other areas to consider are funding, direct or indirect access to affected population, system for managing resources, and accountability and quality control which all depend on the operational modality. *The 5Rs model* that is introduced here outlines the operational modalities of GMH interventions, namely Relief, Response, Recovery, Reinforcement, and Retention. Table 1.2 characterizes each modality as it pertains to GMH work and outlines corresponding objectives for the MH interventions and supports.

Table 1.1 Defining Global Mental Health

Context	International Humanitarian Action
Setting	Humanitarian crisis
	Complex emergency
	Post-conflict recovery
Population needs	Complex needs
Operational modalities or 5Rs	Relief
	Response
	Recovery
	Reinforcement
	Retention

Table 1.2 5Rs Model: Operational Modalities in Global Mental Health

Mode of Operations	*Definition*	*Examples of Interventions*
Relief	Assistance with immediate and imminent needs	Psychological first aid
Response	Response to arising specific issues and addressing their impact, such as an increase in rates of gender-based violence	Psycho-social interventions targeting the specific problems or groups
Recovery	Facilitation and support for sustainable post-conflict recovery	Assisting communities with identifying and mobilizing recovery resources, capacity building (CBPR model)
Reinforcement	Supporting and strengthening the progress, working toward sustainability	Systems and policy development that includes building the referral system Strengthening infrastructure: building and equipping health care and educational facilities
Retention	Retaining the accomplishments Focus on self-reliance Prevention and population management Building resilience towards future destabilizing factors	Capacity building and maintenance Training, ongoing support and professional collaboration with local specialists Peace building

According to the 5Rs model, the role of a GMH and the choice of interventions will be different during immediate disaster relief or when supporting sustainable changes in post-conflict regions because the needs are expected to be different. For example, WHO/mhGAP (2010) outlined the intervention guide for non-specific health settings. There the War Trauma Foundation and World Vision International proposed psychological first aid as the intervention of choice during the relief efforts, further stating that the training of local specialists is crucial for maintaining the recovery gains (WHO/WTF/WVI, 2011). At the same time, the psychological first aid or MHPSS may not be the effective tools for violence prevention and peace building, as it was suggested by Rokhideh (2017) and Bubenzer and Tankink (2017), who called for development of holistic approaches targeting the systems transformation.

Global Mental Health Is Not International Psychology

The humanitarian context that defines GMH distinguishes it from proxy disciplines like international psychology, which primarily focuses on international professional collaborations. The commonly accepted understanding of international psychology is that it is a branch of psychology focusing on the worldwide enterprise of psychology in terms of communication and networking, cross-cultural comparisons, scholarship, practice, and pedagogy (Stevens & Gielen, 2007). Although GMH and international psychology work can overlap, they employ different methodologies to approaching ethics: international psychology works toward establishing the relationship between national psychological associations and developing compatible ethical standards and credentialing of psychologists from different countries (Amstutz, 2013; Leach, Stevens, Lindsay, Ferrero, & Korkut, 2012). The GMH's approach to ethics means developing the values-based framework that integrates professional core values with the universal multidisciplinary values shared by other professionals in humanitarian action (Cherepanov, 2017a).

What's In a Name?

Since its origin GMH has been a battlefield for conflicting views, values, and concepts, both because of its mission and its name. Even the name has become a lightning rod for political and professional controversies: "global" carries negative connotations associated with worries around globalization, "mental health" has embodied concerns around the over-pathologizing paradigm of Western mental health, and finally, the connotation associated with the term mental health may be misleading and stigmatizing because its meaning has little to do with health. I personally have witnessed several good-natured attempts to change the name so it more accurately describes what GMH is about. However, none of them stuck, which was not surprising considering the alternatives: "human response to life adversities" or "human resilience and its failure" and others. Although I agree with the deficiencies and stigma associated with the term GMH, I will use it here for practical reasons, and am open to change whenever a better option becomes available.

Another irony is found in the post hoc efforts to formally define GMH long after the MH professionals had already begun providing services. This was retroactive substantiation of what the professionals had been already practicing and empirically finding beneficial: "I don't care what you call it, I don't care about politically correct terms. It is your job to figure it out why and how it works. I am just doing what makes sense," as one MH professional told me.

1.2 History of Global Mental Health: Quest for Consistency and Standards

In a short period of time, GMH that started as voluntaristic and fragmented efforts by globally minded MH professionals equipped with little but good intentions, has emerged as a professional specialization and managed to establish a highly visible presence in contemporary humanitarian actions. Cherepanov (2016) demonstrated that not only has mainstream MH shaped the concepts of GMH but that GMH reciprocated and has changed the landscape of conventional MH work: global experience has helped to raise awareness of the cultural dimensions in trauma and recovery and to develop appreciation for human resilience.

The historical perspective on GMH allows us to reflect on its past and current struggles, challenges, and accomplishments and identify directions for the future. Although the humanitarian spirit has always drawn people to help those who are in greater need, GMH's origins as a profession can be attributed to three major developments: (a) the inclusion of the PTSD diagnosis in the third edition of the *Diagnostic and Statistical Manual of Mental Disorders* (DSM-III) (APA, 1980), (b) what was at the time a trendy interest in multicultural diversity, and (c) the globalization of humanitarianism. The history of GMH mirrors the major developments in MH and humanitarianism and can be divided into four periods based on the prominent themes: fragmentation, emergence of integrated modules, growth and diversification, and professionalization and accountability. Let us now look into these periods.

1980s: Fragmentation or "the Wild West" of Mental Health

The early 1980s was a pivotal time in trauma psychology, which exploded after the American Psychiatric Association (APA, 1980) added post-traumatic stress disorder (PTSD) to the third edition of its *Diagnostic and Statistical Manual of Mental Disorders* (DSM-III). Although controversial when first introduced, it became an inspiring victory for victims and their advocates. The resultant interest in the clinical and cultural expression of PTSD led professionals to explore the professional frontiers of MH, including the psychological impact of large-scale disasters, genocide, and armed conflicts. Trauma psychology rapidly made major advances, mostly in the area of PTSD symptomatology and epidemiology, both nationally and internationally, which gave impetus to developing trauma treatments.

For example, De Jong, et al. (2001) reported using the Composite International Diagnostic Interview version 2.1 and an adapted version of the Life Events and Social History Questionnaire to study the prevalence of PTSD symptoms in Algeria (37 percent), Cambodia (28 percent), Ethiopia (16 percent), and Gaza (18 percent). They identified specific patterns of risk factors per country, and their findings indicated the importance of contextual differences in the study of traumatic stress and human rights violations.

Unfortunately, fragmented, unregulated, and at times contradictory and even competitive MH interventions lacked consistency and coordination and just added disorganization to the already chaotic situations of complex emergencies. This period demonstrated how the best intentions can become problematic, unethical, risky, and even harmful if they are not supported by professional regulations and standards.

> After the earthquake in Haiti, there were many psychological organizations. They were coming, taking pictures together with us and quickly disappearing without a trace. Sometimes, they were bringing students who were using us as guinea pigs. This didn't feel right. They did not coordinate with each other and every organization was doing whatever they wanted. Sometimes, they were giving us the opposite advice. We did not take them seriously! We wanted to be nice to them but we felt like they were doing this for themselves and not for us. We felt exploited, and ended up going there only if they were giving something to us or children.
>
> (E. Cherepanov, personal communication with a Haitian earthquake survivor, March 18, 2016)

The growing disconnect between trial-and-error interventions and the scarcity of supporting conceptualizations and evidence-based practices in GMH understandably worried the professional community, which by that time had already had established the detrimental impact of unregulated and ethically questionable practices in humanitarian work. This discord demonstrated that, if GMH was to succeed, it had to demonstrate professionalism and overcome the fragmentation of the efforts.

1990s: Integration

The 1990s was a decade of integrated approaches in GMH. The medical and social needs assessments conducted in emergency settings consistently pointed out the complexity of the survivors' needs calling for multidisciplinary interventions. As a result, the psychosocial and integrated primary care models had emerged as the gold standards for the MH supports in emergencies (Cherepanov, 2016).

> Kaz de Jong, the MSF mental health advisor, pointed out that in [a] complex emergency, the mental health and social needs cannot be separated. He questioned, "What do you do if there is enough food, but no one wants to eat?" "Sometimes people are unable to eat because they no longer want to live. They may have witnessed the killing of their family," added De Jong, describing the MH needs during the Bosnian refugee crisis.
>
> (De Jong, 2005)

NGOs expanded the integrated modules targeting special issues like gender-based violence (GBV) and supporting persons with chronic medical conditions, such as HIV, and tuberculosis (TB). The success of the integrated interventions has contributed to establishing multidisciplinary collaborations, shared vision, assessment tools, and protocols that have allowed a move toward primary prevention, and chronic disease and population management. De Jong (2011, p. 5) wrote:

> [S]ince the early 1990s, MSF has implemented psychosocial or mental health interventions in over 40 countries worldwide. The interventions covered various aspects of mental health in different contexts such as acute emergencies, the effects of (acute) trauma, primary healthcare, adaptation and chronic stress-related complaints, psychosocial support to improve outcomes in nutrition, TB and HIV programmes, and psychiatric care in institutions.

Jenkins, Baingana, Ahmad, McDaid, and Atun (2011) believed that integrated approaches are more effective and efficient, and that they would ensure that MH had a budget line and would also allow entry points for MH into other budgets and initiatives. Jenkins et al. (2011) argued that the integration of MH services into primary health care, education, social welfare, social development, and the criminal justice system had a better chance for meeting these complex needs.

The integration trend in GMH did not came out of nowhere. In a way, it mirrored the trend in the mainstream health care that, according to Kodner and Spreeuwenberg (2002), was a counterpoise to its fragmentation. In this day and age, the integrated primary care models have become the approaches of choice in both primary care and behavioral health, and the emergence of a psychosocial integrated model can be traced to the social determinants of health (SDH) approach in community health care (Marmot et al., 2008). The ground assumption is that SDH include socioeconomic status, education, the physical environment, employment, and social support networks as well as access to health care, and that these factors to a large degree determine MH.

The integrated models seems to be gaining edge in different areas of health care and social interventions in GMH as demonstrated by Bubenzer and Tanking (2017), who pointed out the essentiality of integrating MH and psychosocial support with social transformation.

Psychosocial Approaches

In 1996–1999, several leading NGOs—Save the Children, UNICEF, the International Catholic Child Bureau, the International Save the Children Alliance, and Médecins Sans Frontières (MSF)—agreed to designate the psychosocial module as their method of choice (Dagnino, 1996; Save the Children, 1996/2010). And in 2007, the Interagency Standing Committee (IASC) issued their guidelines for MH and psychosocial interventions and support in emergencies (IASC, 2007), which became a major milestone in forming operational standards of GMH. It defined the scope of services and provided guidance for planning and implementing psychosocial interventions as part of multi-sectoral humanitarian relief. The array of roles of GMH providers within the psychosocial approach will be further discussed in Chapter 2.

Integrated Primary Care

The integrated primary care models have been well received by multidisciplinary practitioners. They included co-location, where different services are located in close physical proximity from each other, for instance, in the same building. Souza, Yasuda, and Cristofani (2009), who described the MSF project at Habilla, Darfur, noted that the integration of MH into the primary care system worked well and has been advancing the community's health care (pp. 1–8). Cherepanov (2015a) named other benefits of integrated primary care and MH models in GMH:

- Trauma survivors often suffer from concurrent medical conditions.
- MH services often carry a stigma. Participation in a stand-alone MH program may feel unsafe and stigmatizing for survivors and expose them just by virtue of seeking treatment. On the other hand, receiving medical services is considered to be a much more socially acceptable alternative.
- The integrated model helps to identify "non-medical" sufferers and brings focus to those with more severe impairment.
- Trained primary care providers are able to identify and make referrals for those with MH needs or ambiguous medical conditions. Psychosomatic complaints are often the initial reason to seek a treatment.
- Primary care works as a gateway to MH services. For the survivors of trauma and violence, primary care can often be the only safe option to talk about their experiences.
- An integrated approach assures the continuity of care and the smooth and seamless handoffs between the programs.

When implementing integrated primary care, MH specialists work closely with primary care providers on shared goals, which includes training the health care providers and outreach workers in recognizing the signs of emotional distress so that they can "hand-off" (joined session when MH provider introduces in person), or use other options to refer individuals with higher levels of needs out to the MH services (Kodner & Spreeuwenberg, 2002).

In GMH, the primary care integrated model has demonstrated many advantages, but also revealed its limitations when not supported by concurrent systemic changes. To be sustainable, the interventions and supports must to be backed up by infrastructure development: for instance, helping a victim of intimate partner violence (IPV) is only as effective as the availability of legal, logistics (shelter, finances, employment), aftercare, and community supports. Another example of the systemic complexity is the treatment of HIV or TB, the success of which depends on many interconnected factors, where some are medical, other are psychological (depression affects the treatment adherence), and also social, or logistic (access to medications and testing facilities), including prevention and education.

2000s: Diversification and Policy Development—Quest for Best Practices and Standards of Care

Diversification of Mental Health Programs

In the 2000s, GMH experienced a period of growth and diversification of programs. Cherepanov (2016) provides examples of some GMH programs employed at that time:

- Programs that provide immediate disaster response, trauma treatment in the aftermath of war, famines, and during disease outbreaks: MSF (Kosovo, Bosnia, Sierra Leone, Liberia), SOS Armenia (Armenia), the Haitian Mental Health (HMH) Network.
- Programs geared toward behavioral health aspects of chronic disease or health conditions management including HIV, TB, epilepsy, psychosomatic complaints, ambiguous medical diagnoses, complex needs, and stress and depression that exacerbate health issues and compromise the access to care.
- Maternal and reproductive health, mother and child care, and integrated primary care: MSF (Russia, Tajikistan, Sudan), the Last Mile-Health (Liberia), MDM (Liberia, Syria).
- Programs for victims of violence and gender-based violence: MSF (DRC, Papua New Guinea, and others).
- Programs for special groups—persons with MH disabilities, children, adults, orphans, and others: World Vision, MDM (Liberia), SOS Children's Villages International, Seven Hills International.
- Participation in community development, prevention, education, policy development, training the cadres: Carter Center (Liberia), MDM (long-term development program in the Philippines), Partners in Health (Haiti).

The proliferation of MH programs revealed the dearth of evidenced-based practices and outcome measures, which put pressure on GMH to demonstrate its usefulness to donors, beneficiaries, and the professional community. Mollica et al. (2004, pp. 2058–2067) underscored the need for standardized approaches to the assessment thereof, monitoring the outcomes of which is crucial to evidence-driven quality improvement, and the dissemination of the results achieved. To the layman, the element of mystery often surrounding the psychological work for some time deferred inquiries about the programmatic choices as to why specific models and methods were being used and not others. This created a paradoxical situation where, while the NGOs mainly embraced the importance of MH work, the added value largely remained unclear. "I am so glad that mental health people finally arrived. We needed you so much because you always carry condoms!" With these exact words a project director once greeted me (E. Cherepanov, personal communication, August 10, 1999). With the difficulties of demonstrating the effectiveness of MH interventions, the professional community and donors continued to press the question of its overall impact. Additionally, the lack of guidelines, standards and regulations complicated the development of systems of complementary interventions and delayed the GMH integration into humanitarian action, where the humanitarian response is as effective as it is consistent, coordinated, and collaborative.

Policy Developments

The breakthrough for the emerging role of GMH on the humanitarian stage came in 2000–2001, after the World Health Organization (WHO) declared MH a global priority and issued a report that highlighted the crucial role of MH in the overall well-being of individuals, societies, and countries (WHO, 2001). The report advocated for changes in global policies that were urgently needed to ensure that the stigma and discrimination of MH issues were broken down, and that effective prevention and MH treatment were put into place. As a follow-up, the Mental Health Global Action Plan (WHO/mhGAP, 2010) outlined strategic and tactical priorities for GMH to improve the MH of diverse populations. Its essence is in building partnerships for collective action and reinforcing the commitment of governments, international organizations, and other stakeholders. Since then, the WHO has undertaken various projects, such as the Global Campaign Against Epilepsy and the Global Campaign for Suicide Prevention, with a focus on scaling up services for mental, neurological, and substance use disorders especially for low- and middle-income countries.

In implementing the mhGAP strategic directions, the Interagency Standing Committee (IASC, 2007) developed the guidelines for mental health and psychosocial supports (MHPSS) in emergencies. These established the operational framework for psychosocial interventions, which became a milestone in the paradigmatic development of GMH. Another important step was the Movement for Global Mental Health (MGMH), which was formed in 2008 to raise the profile of the neglected agenda of MH in the world and to be a global platform for sharing ideas and empirical findings. The movement was vocal in raising concerns about ethically problematic areas, especially in defining its agenda (MGMH, 2014).

2010–Present: Professionalization and Accountability

In September of 2015, the United Nations (UN) included the MH module in their sustainable development goals (SDGs). In this historic step, the UN acknowledged the burden of disease and designated MH as a priority for global development over the next 15 years. The currently acting Comprehensive Mental Health Action Plan 2013–2020 (WHO/mhGAP, 2008) calls for a change in attitudes that perpetuate stigma and discrimination against mental illness, as well as for the expansion of services to promote greater efficiency in the use of resources.

The growing gap between GMH undertaking more ambitious tasks and the tidal wave of criticism of its agenda signaled the need to align its methodology with the latest professional developments and to identify problematic areas requiring future consideration. That is why it almost came as no surprise when Minas, Wright, and Kakuma (2014) and Eaton, Kakuma, Wright, and Minas (2014) proclaimed that the movement for GMH was in transition (i.e. in crisis), which meant the time had come to reflect on its goals and on the form of organizational structure that would best serve the GMH mission. This self-proclaimed crisis was yet another indication of the synchronicity of processes in modern humanitarianism when the emerging themes were professionalization of humanitarian response, accountability, and quality assurance (Sphere, 2004, 2014). In response to the challenges of globalization and industrialization of humanitarianism, the humanitarian community has launched a number of initiatives to improve quality and performance (Sphere, 2004). Influenced by these processes, GMH has been focusing on establishing standards of practice and professional competencies where the development of an ethical framework is envisioned as an important step in this overarching agenda.

It is worth noting that the holistic approach has been getting professional attention as a direction for the future. The proponents of this approach propose development and implementation of cross-sectional models that would allow addressing the mind–body–social–spiritual connection as a whole (Ng et al., 2009). The approach stems from the dissatisfaction with limitations of the cross-sectional silos partitioning the responses to complex needs and proposes multilayer, multimodal, and cross-sectional interventions, unified under the umbrella of the peace-building agenda (Bubenzer & Tankink, 2017). Table 1.3 describes the major milestones in the formation of the humanitarian values as they pertain to GMH.

Table 1.3 History of Global Mental Health

Timetable	*Name*	*Characteristics*	*Major Developments*
1980s	Fragmentation or best intentions	Interventions are fragmented, uncoordinated, and driven mostly by the provider's best intentions without regard for the population needs or professional accountability Experimentation and use of tools with questionable validity and unclear effectiveness	1980: inclusion of PTSD into DSM-III Growing interest in PTSD and its epidemiology Questioning cultural validity of PTSD Trial and error experimentation with different approaches and interventions
1990s	Integration and emergence of integrated modules	The multidisciplinary interventions help to address complex needs Psychosocial and integrated primary care models	1992: the IASC was established in response to UN Resolution 46/182 on the strengthening of humanitarian assistance. General Assembly Resolution 48/57 affirmed its role as the primary mechanism for inter-agency coordination of humanitarian assistance

(*continued*)

Table 1.3 (Cont.)

Timetable	*Name*	*Characteristics*	*Major Developments*
2000s	Growth and diversification	Proliferation of GMH Quest for consistency, professional standards, and best practices Critique	2000: UN declared MH a global priority 2008/2010: WHO/mhGAP called for scaling-up services for mental, neurological, and substance use disorders especially for low- and middle-income countries 2007: *IASC Guidelines on Mental Health and Psychosocial Support in Emergency Settings* 2008: Movement for Global Mental Health (MGMH) was formed to raise the profile of the neglected agenda of MH in the world and to be a global platform for sharing ideas and empirical findings. Its critique of the movement laid out the directions for the future development
2010–present	Professionalization and accountability Population management Holistic approaches Peace building	Main themes: professionalization of humanitarian action, humanitarian accountability, establishing standards of practice, quality assurance, and cross-sectional and holistic interventions	2010: Grand Challenges in global mental health: a consortium of researchers, advocates, and clinicians announces its research priorities for improving the lives of people with mental illness around the world, and calls for urgent action and investment

1.3 Controversies and the Grand Challenges

Controversies

Controversies have been plaguing GMH since its origin, and it has had to work hard to prove its viability. Locke's stirring statement is indicative to this apprehensive attitude:

> as "global health" is consolidated as an interdisciplinary field of inquiry and intervention, flush with new money and motivation to address disparities in disease burden and inadequate or ailing health systems, mental health researchers and professionals have been working to advocate for the importance of what they have taken to calling "global mental health," drawing on burden of disease problematic data.
>
> (Locke, 2015, p. 194)

By being at the crossroads of the development of MH, the humanitarian movement, and globalism, GMH has opened itself to transformative global processes and the associated "war of paradigms" reflecting the conceptual disagreements within both the professional community and the humanitarian movement. The critique of GMH mainly extended in three directions: (a) the validity of Western MH concepts, (b) the contextual relevance of its methods, and (c) its mission.

GMH, despite its growing pains, has been able to assert its vital role in the humanitarian action and has managed to turn this battlefield into a proving ground for concept development. This critique spotlighted the fundamental problems with the biomedical paradigm of MH and strengthened advocacy for paradigmatic changes in the mainstream MH. The methodology of research, assessment, and treatment tools for PTSD and depression was called into question over concerns of pathologizing normal human reactions to life adversities and the problematic cross-cultural validity of Western diagnoses (Hinton & Lewis-Fernandez, 2011; Patel, 2001; Yehuda & McFarlane, 2009). If not addressed, the medicalization of suffering, iatrogenic effects, and misuse of psychiatric medications threatened to undermine the mission of GMH as these bring more harm than good (Summerfield, 1999, 2004, 2012). Summerfield voiced concerns that exporting psychiatric paradigms of treatment may irreversibly alter the MH care systems of the developing world. Patel (2014), who advocated for the universality of the Western diagnoses of certain mental illness, agreed that others categories, such as depression in particular, do not travel well across cultures and that the use of such labels represents a medicalization of a social condition where the solutions lie not within a medical approach but more likely within the social or political sphere.

The evaluation of the effectiveness of interventions also became an area of contention due to problematic cross-cultural transferability of evidence-based outcomes measures. A thorough desk review of existing psychosocial assessments and evaluations done by the Mailman School of Public Health (2009, p. 3) identified a number of widespread problems in GMH that led to questionable or inconclusive results, including:

- lack of clear and appropriate project objectives;
- a number of common methodological weaknesses in evaluations;

- lack of appropriate and standardized quantitative tools for assessing psychosocial well-being. The strengths and weaknesses of the available tools lie in the cultural validity of underlying concepts and disagreements about what can be considered a good outcome.

Kirmayer and Pedersen (2014) expressed concerns that the WHO and other allies have become too focused on developing, implementing, and evaluating evidence-based practices, and proposed that the goal could be shifted to improving access to services or interventions and reducing the global treatment gap for mental disorders to better match the GMH mission.

> Recent debates on global mental health have raised questions about the goals and consequences of current approaches. Some of these critiques emphasize the difficulties and potential dangers of applying Western categories, concepts, and interventions given the ways that culture shapes illness experience. The concern is that in the urgency to address disparities in global health, interventions that are not locally relevant and culturally consonant will be exported with negative effects including inappropriate diagnoses and interventions, increased stigma, and poor health outcomes. More fundamentally, exclusive attention to mental disorders identified by psychiatric nosologies may shift attention from social structural determinants of health that are among the root causes of global health disparities.
>
> (Kirmayer & Pedersen, 2014, p. 759)

But the core point of contention became the concept of the "burden of the disease" itself, which was used to argue that mental illness constitutes a "hidden epidemic" in poor countries. As the burden of the disease became a driving force behind the policy development of GMH, including prioritizing research, funding, and the practice development, the integrity of the supporting data came into question in two directions: Patel et al. (2007) suggested that we cannot really differentiate the impact of MH from other factors such as poor health or poverty. Even more controversial became the disability adjusted life years (DALYs) metric used in the study (Murray, 1994). Anand & Hanson (1997) further voiced concerns about using the same measure for both assessing health status and the resources allocation purposes because this would be "mixing up health and economics." But the main objections came from the disability advocates who fiercely disputed the underlying assumption that if we measure the quality of life by years of healthy life and not by its quality, this perpetuates the stigmatization of disability and devalues the life of a disable person.

Concerns about the impact of globalization on vulnerable populations amplified the worries that GMH can be used as an agent of influence. The critics saw in GMH, and especially in psychiatric treatment, a form of neocolonialism and a setback in the larger trend of de-pathologizing psychological trauma. The proponents of the psychosocial approach labeled the very term "mental health" as misleading because of its inherently pathological connotation and suggested instead a focus on normal human reactions to life adversities (E. Cherepanov, personal communication, October 18, 2013). The critical voices became particularly persuasive after Summerfield's (1999) infectious critique of assumptions behind psychological trauma programs in war-affected areas, where he cautioned against using the biomedical model of suffering for pharmaceutical companies' profits. Watters, an avid critic of GMH, added to these controversies with his unambiguously titled book, *Crazy Like Us: The Globalization of the American Psyche*. He went on to claim that GMH was a product of American-led globalization and that "a loose group of anthropologists and cross-cultural psychiatrists" have for many years been busily engaged in a grand project of Americanizing the world's understanding of MH and illness, which carries a political agenda (Watters, 2010a, 2010b). In the midst of these controversies, Patel and Prince's (2010) definition of GMH as a tool for "improving mental health and achieving equity in mental health for all people worldwide" added fuel to the fire. This definition seemed to further imply that GMH's mission is to "improve" MH in a way aligned with how Westerners understand it (see Figure 1.1). It was just a matter of time before pushback could be expected, and in 2013, China Mills published the book *Decolonizing Global Mental*

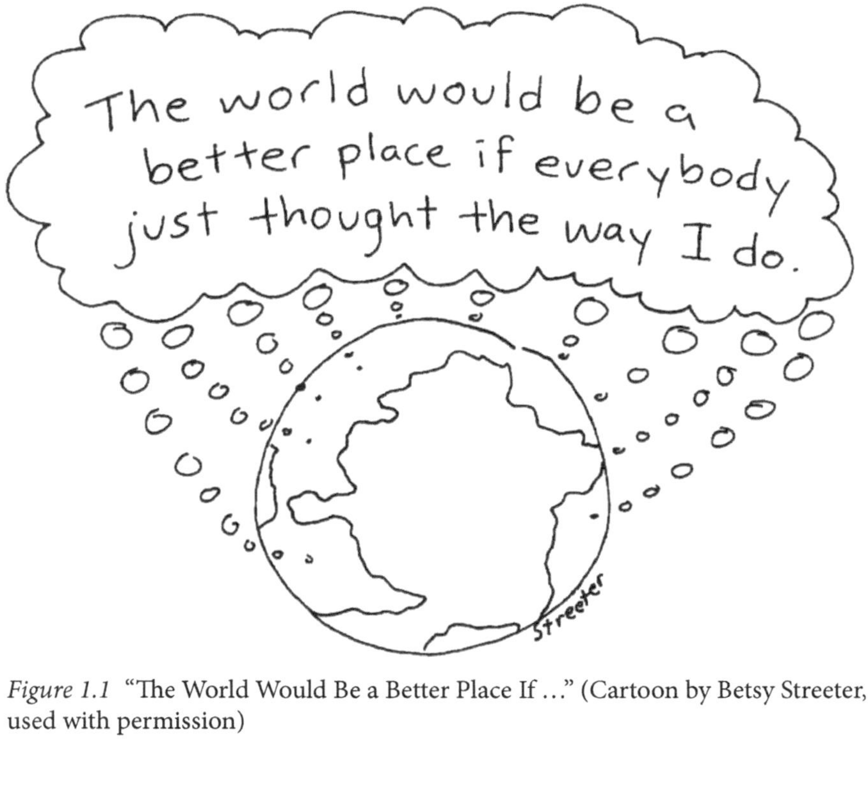

Figure 1.1 "The World Would Be a Better Place If…" (Cartoon by Betsy Streeter, used with permission)

Health: The Psychiatrization of the Majority World. In this book and in an interview with the Movement for Global Mental Health newsletter (MGMH, 2014), Mills (2013) shared her belief that GMH is a "neocolonial" or "missionary" project and was furthermore primarily a front for pharmaceutical companies seeking new clients for psychiatric drugs—that GMH was a form of neocolonialism "swallowed in the form of a pill." According to Mills' interview, the GMH view of the world painted an anxious space where socioeconomic crises came to be reconfigured as individual crises—as "mental illness"—and how potentially violent interventions came to be seen as "essential" treatment. This criticism underscored the pressing need of the values, regulations, and professional competencies in GMH. The same critique became a driving force behind professional self-determination, accountability, and establishing professional standards—and, frankly, the writing of this book.

Grand Challenges Initiative

To respond to criticism, the National Institute of Mental Health (NIMH) and the Global Alliance for Chronic Disease, in partnership with the Welcome Trust, the McLaughlin-Rotman Centre for Global Health, and the London School of Hygiene and Tropical Medicine, launched the Grand Challenges in Global Mental Health initiative to identify the top challenges and focus the professional collective efforts on addressing these challenges:

> The identified challenges captured three broad themes. First, the results underscore the need for research that uses a life-course approach. Second, the challenges recognize that the suffering caused by mental and neurological disorders extends beyond the patient to family members and communities. Third, the challenges underline the fact that all care and treatment interventions—psychosocial or pharmacological, simple or complex—should have an evidence base to provide programme planners, clinicians, and policymakers with effective care packages.
>
> (Collins et al., 2011, p. 28)

The panel underscored important relationships between environmental exposures and MH disorders. It concluded that extreme poverty, war, and natural disasters affect large swathes of the world, and we still do not fully understand the mechanisms by which mental disorders might be averted or precipitated in those settings. The Initiative called for urgent action and investment in GMH where the main theme was the need for global cooperation in the conduct of research to create shared access to data, expertise, and capacity-building opportunities, and where children emerged as requiring particular attention for prevention and care.

CHAPTER 2

Contemporary Humanitarianism

2.1 Understanding Contemporary Humanitarianism and its Challenges

> Idealism increases in direct proportion to one's distance from the problem.
> (John Galsworthy, cited in Larkey & Devereux, 1999, p. 170)

To better understand the changing role of GMH in the complex realities of modern-day humanitarianism, this chapter reviews the history of humanitarian values and the arising controversies, and examines the emerging trends and challenges to the humanitarian agenda. While the significance of humanitarianism is never in question, its principles and values continue to develop along with increasing understanding of the complexity and changeability of the humanitarian action—and also exposing its limitations.

Humanitarianism refers to the practice of saving lives, alleviating suffering, and promoting human welfare. The World Health Organization (WHO) defines humanitarian action as "the assistance, protection, and advocacy actions undertaken on an impartial basis in response to human needs resulting from complex emergencies and natural hazards" (Glossary of Humanitarian Terms, 2008, p. 31).

The very term "humanitarian" is associated with caring, compassion, and "feeling good." A closer look, however, reveals its complexity and opens it up to difficult questions such as those about politicizing aid, which have been incredibly damaging for the movement. These lingering controversies have been eroding the idea of humanitarian aid, compromising the mission of NGOs, and putting aid workers and beneficiaries at risk. As Noam Chomsky argued, "for one thing, there's a history of humanitarian intervention. You can look at it. And when you do, you discover that virtually every use of military force is described as humanitarian intervention" (cited in Jayakumar, 2012).

Nicholas de Torrente, former executive director of MSF-USA, discusses the connection between politicization of humanitarianism and the safety of aid workers in his paper "Humanitarian Action Under Attack," where he described this dilemma as a double bind: How do humanitarians continue to reach people in need when the Western policy makers want to assimilate them into their political and military agendas on the one hand, and anti-Western extremists want to kill them on the other (de Torrente, 2004, p. 2)? De Torrente went on to conclude that in order to continue saving lives and relieving human suffering, humanitarians can and should rediscover their roots, i.e. humanitarian values that are apolitical by nature and prove themselves politically neutral, impartial, and independent. He suggests that these fundamental humanitarian principles serve two essential purposes. They embody humanitarian ideals of alleviating suffering, unconditionally and without any ulterior motive. Their adoption helps in obtaining both the consent of belligerents and the trust of communities for the presence and activities of humanitarian organizations, particularly in highly volatile contexts:

> The most important principles of humanitarian action are humanity, which posits the conviction that all people have equal dignity by virtue of their membership in humanity; impartiality, which directs that assistance is provided based solely on need, without discrimination among recipients; neutrality, which stipulates that humanitarian organizations must refrain from taking part in hostilities or taking actions that advantage one side of the conflict over another; and independence, which is necessary to ensure that humanitarian action only serves the interests of war victims, and not political, religious, or other agendas.
>
> (de Torrente, 2004, pp. 5–6)

His opponents argued that either humanitarian aid cannot be fully insulated from politics (Abiew, 2012) or that humanitarianism may not be an appropriate instrument to further protection of vulnerable populations (Rieff, 2002).

2.2 History of Humanitarian Values

The history of humanitarian values offers insight into its present-day challenges and trends as it has mirrored the struggle of the humanitarian community to establish consistency in multidisciplinary interventions where the measure of success is saving human lives and alleviating suffering.

The humanitarian activities during World War II demonstrated the need for universal values based on humanitarian law, and in 1848, the General Assembly of the United Nations (UN) adopted the Universal Declaration of Human Rights. This Declaration was the first global expression of what many people believe to be the rights to which all human beings are inherently entitled, and it committed all member states to promote "universal respect for, and observance of, human rights and fundamental freedoms for all without distinction as to race, sex, language, or religion" (UNGA, 1948). In the first four years post-World War II, as Rysaback-Smith (2015) pointed out, there was a sudden and unprecedented growth of non-governmental organizations (NGOs). Over 200 organizations were established, which became a cornerstone for the development of humanitarianism as we know it. Aid became more global with increasing advances in transportation and communication and began to shift from Europe to the less developed parts of the world. This growth and diversification of humanitarian action brought to the forefront the need for shared values, consistency, and coordination of operations. Not all the developments in humanitarian action have direct relevance to GMH, and Table 2.1 summarizes the historical milestones that have proven most essential to forming the system of values governing GMH.

- *1965.* The twentieth conference of the International Federation of the Red Cross and Red Crescent societies adopted the fundamental principles of the movement: humanity, impartiality, neutrality, independence, voluntary service, unity, and universality. These principles have become integral to the development of humanitarianism, serving both as a guide for action and the movement's common identity and purpose (IFRC, 1965).
- *1960–1970s.* The Biafran Civil War (Nigeria), during which civilians were murdered and starved by blockading forces, spotlighted controversies around humanitarian neutrality in armed conflicts or during genocides. The disagreement around this principle led to the formation of Médecins Sans Frontières (MSF) when Recamier and Kouchner, the founders of MSF, envisioned a form of humanitarianism that would ignore political or religious boundaries in favor of prioritizing the welfare of those suffering. They believed the world needed to know about the events they were witnessing and proposed that solidarity replace the neutrality principle (MSF, 1971).
- *1980s.* The massive impact of media exposure during periods of Ethiopian famine revealed shortfalls of uncoordinated and disorganized humanitarian response. The inefficiency, fragmentation, and duplications of the relief efforts led to the interdisciplinary initiatives from which the Sphere Project (1997) and IASC Project (2007) later emerged. A growing body of evidence has emphasized the importance of coordination and standards of work.
- *1990s.* Scholars labeled the 1990s as a "decade of humanitarian military interventions," during which the UN authorized several interventions on humanitarian grounds (Kaldor, 2007, p. 16), which extremely disturbed the humanitarian community concerned about diluting the meaning of humanitarianism (Jayakumar, 2012) and increasing risks for aid workers (de Torrente, 2004).
- *1990.* The situation in post-genocide Rwanda polarized humanitarian actors and challenged some of the ground principles of humanitarian response, such as whether to provide humanitarian aid to those who perpetrated genocide. Storey (1997) noted that this dilemma prompted the renewed discussions about the values and limits of humanitarian action.
- *1991.* The United Nations established OCHA, the Office for the Coordination of Humanitarian Affairs, to bring together humanitarian actors and ensure a coherent response to emergencies. OCHA's mission is to mobilize and coordinate humanitarian action and to promote the humanitarian community's compliance with humanitarian principles in every humanitarian response (UN/OCHA, 1991).

- *1992.* The United Nations (UN) and NGOs initiated a number of initiatives and collaborative partnerships designed to strengthen the response to complex emergencies and natural disasters, while improving the overall effectiveness of humanitarian operations in the field as well as their accountability. The UN General Assembly resolution 46/182 established IASC, the Interagency Standing Committee, a primary mechanism for interagency coordination of humanitarian assistance. It is a unique forum involving key UN and non-UN humanitarian partners (UN/IASC, 1992).
- *1994.* Eight of the world's largest disaster relief NGOs adopted the NGO Code of Conduct, which sets up consistent conduct expectations from humanitarian workers (Code of Conduct, 1994).
- *1997.* The UN and NGOs initiated a number of initiatives and collaborative partnerships aiming to improve accountability of the humanitarian system in disaster response, out of which emerged the Sphere Project (1997), which was charged with developing minimum standards in core areas of humanitarian assistance and enhancing their accountability (Sphere Project, 2004). The Sphere Project:
  - summarized standards of quality and accountability for humanitarian response;
  - affirmed principles of the humanitarian imperative, which is that action should be taken to prevent or alleviate human suffering arising out of disaster or conflict, and that nothing should override this principle;
  - affirmed core legal principles that have the most bearing on the welfare of those affected by disaster or conflict.
- *2000s.* The "war on terrorism" was a name for the international military campaign that was launched by the US and UK governments and their allies after the September 1, 2011 attacks in the United States (Schmitt & Shanker,). The "war on terrorism" has made the environment even more dangerous for humanitarians and brought attention to their safety and MH needs.
- *2002.* In the wake of the "aid for sex" scandals, and amid the allegations of sexual abuse of refugees by peacekeepers and aid workers in West Africa, Congo, Kosovo, and Haiti (Dodds, 2017; Jordan, 2004; Nichols, 2016), the IASC proclaimed the humanitarian commitment to actively prevent and respond to sexual exploitation and abuse by humanitarian workers, and to implement this commitment in all humanitarian response operations. They reaffirmed their determination to eradicate acts of sexual exploitation and abuse by their personnel and to actively respond to incidents that are perpetuated against their beneficiaries (IASC, 2015).
- *2007.* The IASC published the *Guidelines on Mental Health and Psychosocial Support in Emergency Settings* (IASC, 2007), issuing strategic guidance for MH and trauma intervention modules in GMH.
- *2016.* The first ever World Humanitarian Summit (WHS, 2016), which took place in Istanbul on May 23–24, 2016, was a global call to action to fundamentally reform the humanitarian aid industry to react more effectively to today's many crises. The Summit had three main goals:

1. To re-inspire and reinvigorate a commitment to humanity and to the universality of humanitarian principles.
2. To initiate a set of concrete actions and commitments aimed at enabling countries and communities to better prepare for and respond to crises and be resilient to shocks.
3. To share best practices that can help save lives around the world, put affected people at the center of humanitarian action, and alleviate suffering.

The Summit Outcomes

- Prioritized education in humanitarian action and set up the "Education Cannot Wait" fund (UNICEF, 2016).
- Established the Charter on Inclusion of Persons with Disabilities in Humanitarian Action, which was hailed as "a victory for disabled people who have been largely ignored in humanitarian aid operations" (Handicap International, 2016).
- Launched the first ever global compact to address the needs of youth in crisis settings (WHS, 2016).
- Critique by NGOs:
    - NGOs called for a shift of power and funding from international organizations to those working on the ground. Currently, local organizations receive 2 percent of direct humanitarian funding, with the rest going to organizations based in Europe and the United States (Wall, 2016).
    - Expressed concern that the Summit disproportionately focused on the incorporation of humanitarian assistance into a broader development and resilience agenda while neglecting emergency response, particularly in conflict areas or epidemic situations (Goldberg, 2016).
    - Found it unacceptable that adapting humanitarian action to the differing needs tailored to gender, age, and disability was not being given high enough priority (Oxfam, 2016).
    - Regretfully, the issue of safety and well-being of the aid workers "did not appear to have gained any prominence" at the Summit (Maudling, 2016).

The beautiful graphic pictograms illustrate three out of the Seven Fundamental Principles of the Red Cross Movement (from the Namibia Red Cross webpage: www.redcross.int/EN/fundprincips/namibiaseven.asp)

2.3 Emerging Trends in Humanitarian Action: Professionalization and Accountability

Emerging Trends

Over the past decade, the humanitarian community has been facing unprecedented challenges: according to the United Nations High Commission for Refugees

Table 2.1 Abbreviated History of Humanitarian Values

Year	*Organizations and Events*	*Key Developments and Impact*
1948	The United Nations (UN) General Assembly	Universal Declaration of Human Rights
1965	The 20th International Conference of the Red Cross and Red Crescent	Fundamental principles of the movement: humanity, impartiality, independence, and neutrality
1971	The Biafran Civil War (Nigeria)	Principle of neutrality is challenged Formation of Médecins Sans Frontières (MSF)
1980s	Ethiopian famine	Global awareness of shortfalls of humanitarian action. Call for consistency and coordination in humanitarian action
1991	The Office for Coordination of Humanitarian Affairs (UN/ OCHA)	Established to mobilize and coordinate humanitarian action and to promote the humanitarian community's compliance with humanitarian principles in every humanitarian response
1994	The International Federation of Red Cross and Red Crescent Societies (IFRC)	NGOs' Code of Conduct sets up consistent conduct expectations from humanitarian workers
1997	The Sphere Project	Developed a set of minimum standards in core areas of humanitarian assistance to enhance the accountability of the humanitarian system in disaster response
2000s	"Aid for sex" scandal	Prompted stance against sexual exploitation and abuse
2007	The Inter-Agency Standing Committee (IASC) Guidelines	*Guidelines on Mental Health and Psychosocial Support in Emergency Settings* (IASC, 2007)
May, 2016	The World Humanitarian Summit (WHS)	Delivered a global call to action to fundamentally reform the humanitarian aid industry to react more effectively to today's many crises

(UNHCR, n.d.) data, the worst refugee crisis since World War II now counts more than 50 million worldwide, and as of June 2015, one in every 122 people had been displaced by war, violence, or persecution. In Syria alone, there are upwards of 7.6 million internally displaced persons. In response to overwhelming needs, the humanitarian relief has expanded its presence: Lewis (2014) and Riddell (2008) believed that more than 35,000 international NGOs and millions of national NGOs exist worldwide. Rysaback-Smith (2015) went on to state that massive proliferation of humanitarian assistance has led to both positive and negative developments in aid provision and will likely continue to greatly impact the ground values of delivery of aid far into the future. When introducing standards for their humanitarian charter, the Sphere Project described the current trends in humanitarian relief as such:

- Humanitarianism has widened from purely charitable "philanthropy" to include rights-based and professional approaches.
- Advocacy with governments has been more common in recent times.
- There is an increasing need to accept that conflicts are chronic in some developing countries.
- Principles are needed to keep humanitarian work separate from militaries and politics.
- Disasters are increasingly complex and require complex approaches.
- There is increasing diversity in the humanitarian community.
- There is increasing complexity of organizations involved in operating (Sphere, 2004, p. 10).

Shifting Strategic Priorities: Emphasis on Development

Mackintosh (2000) inferred that the main trend in the modern era of humanitarianism has been a shift in thinking from short-term aid provision and immediate mitigation of suffering to developmental aid largely provided by so-called

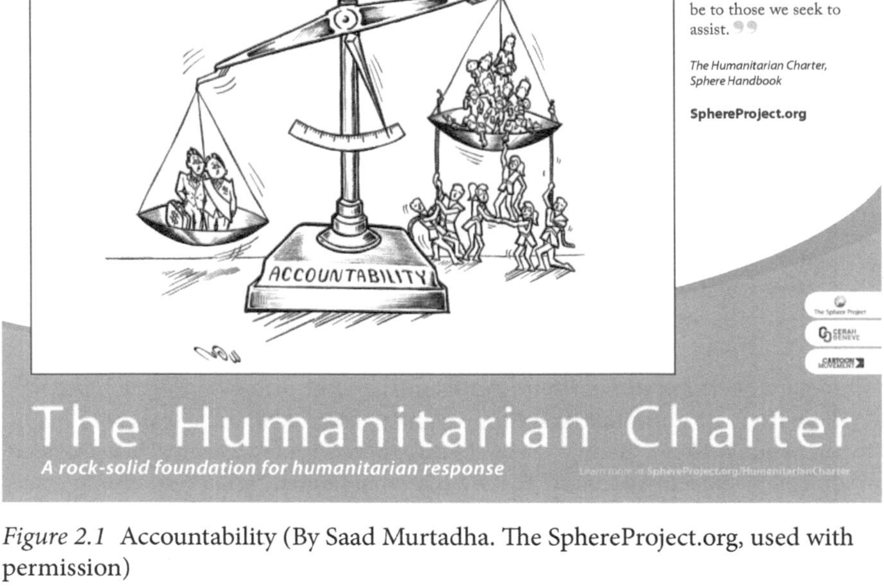

Figure 2.1 Accountability (By Saad Murtadha. The SphereProject.org, used with permission)

developed countries. This trend also points to a potential shift in global political and governmental interest and funding from as-needed provision of assistance to a long-term and complex developmental strategy, which accentuated the always delicate balance between cost-effectiveness and humanitarian ideology. This trend was clearly reflected in the outcomes of the World Humanitarian Summit (WHS) in 2016, which was criticized for neglecting the immediate needs of populations during wars, famines, or epidemics (WHS, 2016).

Globalization of Humanitarianism

The severity and complexity of current and ongoing humanitarian crises having global impacts necessitated increased interaction of aid providers through the growth of the international flow of money, resources, logistics, ideas, and culture. At the same time, the globalization processes revealed that the perceived universality of the humanitarian agenda can collide with sovereignty-based and nationalistic discourses. This process seems to be reinforced by the emergence of non-Western responses to disasters (Islamic NGOs, new donors from the Gulf, etc.) (Donini, n.d.; Global Journal, n.d.), and in several countries there has been backlash against humanitarian action from government officials, the media, religious groups, and portions of civil society. In the paper "Can Globalization Transform Humanitarian Aid," Moran (2010) warned that globalization was enabling conflicts and their destabilizing consequences to be "exported" in the form of economic instability and political unrest, which required adjustment in humanitarian strategies:

> The increasingly complex nature of conflict in the world today demands a … response that is globally oriented yet also takes into account local histories and circumstances. In the face of ever-increasing war, conflict, and development challenges, strengthened regional and international cooperation and increased "buy-in" from actors at all levels of society is critical in ensuring a robust humanitarian response. Such a response must meet both current and future needs of at-risk populations; only then will we be able to fully provide the necessary social protections for vulnerable communities and address new challenges as they arise. Globalization, itself a source of transformative change, necessitates the implementation of a relief strategy that is equally transformative. By capitalizing on our increased connectivity, we can best address the increasingly complex humanitarian challenges we face.

Professionalization of Humanitarianism: Humanitarian Action as Industry

Walker, Hein, Russ, Bertleff, and Caspers (2010) asserted that the scale of humanitarian action makes it an industry that must operate professionally. They provided a somewhat shocking account: The international humanitarian response to crises employs 210,000 people and accounts for nearly $15 billion in spending globally each year. They further suggested that we should no longer regard humanitarian work as driven by best intentions alone, especially in the medical or health care related sectors, but rather as an industry that requires professionalization. Walker et al. (2010, p. 2224) further argue that

> aid workers operate through organizations that have grown in size and complexity to match the increase in the populations served. The big aid agencies of today are transnational, multimillion- or even multibillion-dollar not-for-profit corporations. Inevitably in such a growth market, a plethora of new actors has emerged, including small local NGOs; mega-churches and mega-mosques, each of which provides millions of dollars of assistance; and military operations that have blurred the line between campaigns for civilians' hearts and minds and traditional humanitarian aid. Thus, today's aid workers must operate in a far more complex and more challenging environment, over far longer periods of time, than their predecessors did.

Walker et al. (2010) went on to outline challenges to the professionalization of humanitarian aid where workers face different barriers, including gaining access to training, paying for it, and the lack of universally accepted credentials. Workers, aid organizations, and the training programs alike have no way to evaluate, use, or benefit from a coherent career path in which new experiences fit into or build on prior knowledge to create a portfolio. The authors recommended developing professional associations and offered a list of competencies and core professional knowledge for professional aid workers.

The conclusion was that core professional knowledge areas of any professional actors such as GMH, must include understanding the structure of the humanitarian sector; having a firm grasp of international humanitarian law and refugee law; understanding basic safety and security issues; and being aware of the mandates and principles of the key humanitarian organizations. The concentration on professionalism would improve accountability and make the provision of humanitarian aid more evidence-based, reflecting exactly what has happened in the field of medicine. This is expected to strengthen the links between university-based research programs and agencies' practices, leading to more appropriate aid and more knowledge about the true impact that aid has on at-risk populations.

Quality and Accountability: Using Power Responsibly

The 1994 Rwanda genocide, the 2004 Asian tsunami, the 2010 Haiti earthquake, and other major crises put accountability and the quality of humanitarian interventions at the top of our list of priorities (see Figure 2.1). Lloyd, Blagescu, and de las Casa (2005, p. 5) saw in accountability "the processes through which an organization makes a commitment to respond to and balance the needs of stakeholders in its decision-making processes and activities, and delivers against this commitment." The commitment to humanitarian accountability led to establishing in 2003 the Humanitarian Accountability Partnership International

(HAP International) (Jordan & van Tuijl, 2006, p. 39). This multi-agency initiative works to improve the accountability and responsibility of global organizations, and to strengthen the capacity of civil society to better engage in decision-making processes. The responsible use of power means that survivors of war or disaster must be able to influence decisions about the help they receive, and they can give feedback and complain if they feel the "helping power" was not exercised well. Lloyd et al.'s (2005) reflection on accountability suggested that global processes had demonstrated that NGO accountability systems were skewed toward those stakeholders with the most power and influence. As a solution, the movement for accountability proposed that giving voice and engaging beneficiaries in decision-making would provide them with a platform for participation that would increase both effectiveness and learning. This position can be summarized as "Nothing about us without us," a slogan that initially had been used in a disability rights context to communicate the idea that no policy should be decided without representation including the full and direct participation of members of the group(s) affected by that policy (Charlton, 1998; UN Chronicle, 2004).

CHAPTER 3
Humanitarian Ethics

3.1 Humanitarian Charter: Minimum Standards for Humanitarian Response

This chapter examines the role of the Humanitarian Charter and the NGO Code of Conduct in establishing the cross-sectional standards and values to govern multidisciplinary operations to assure, as has been shown in the previous chapter, the coordinated multidisciplinary and cross-sectional collaborations.

The critical importance of consistent and coordinated interventions and the shared standards became apparent in the aftermath of the catastrophic level of death during Ethiopian famines in 1983–1985. The Rwanda genocide in 1994 highlighted the core problem stemming from the neutrality proclaimed by NGOs, who offered supports to the genocidal regime of Rwanda (Storey, 1997, p. 384) raising the concern that the faithful following of the humanitarian principle of neutrality was equated with support of the regime. The genocide against the Tutsi took place in the context of the Rwandan Civil War, which was a genocidal mass slaughter of Tutsi in Rwanda by members of the Hutu majority government. An estimated 500,000 to 1,000,000 Rwandans were killed during the 100-day period from April 7 to mid-July 1994, constituting as many as 70 percent of the Tutsi population (Mark, 2009; Orbinski, 2009).

The followed massive media exposure revealed the inadequacy of humanitarian action to protect populations and spotlighted another issue, which was the chaotic, fragmented, and inefficient interventions. In response, the Sphere Project (1997, 2004) was set up to develop minimum standards in core areas of humanitarian assistance to improve the quality of assistance provided to people affected by disasters, and to enhance the accountability of the humanitarian system in disaster response. In collaboration with leading NGOs, interested donor governments, and UN agencies, the Sphere Project developed a Handbook of the Humanitarian Charter and Minimum Standards, aimed to both disseminate the resultant products widely throughout the international humanitarian system and to encourage their formal adoption and practice by relief agencies and their donors. The Handbook, which was adopted by participating NGOs, established minimum standards for humanitarian chapters, including coordination, evaluations, operational research, and training (Sphere, 2014).

This Humanitarian Charter or the cornerstone of the Sphere Project is built upon the principles and provisions of international humanitarian law, international human rights law, refugee law, and the Code of Conduct for the International Red Cross and Red Crescent Movement and NGOs in Disaster Relief. The Charter describes the core principles that govern humanitarian action and asserts the right of populations to protection and assistance. The Health Action section of the Charter recognizes the horrors, losses, uncertainties, and numerous other stressors associated with conflict and other disasters that place people at increased risk of diverse social, behavioral, psychological, and psychiatric problems. It positions MH and psychosocial work as an essential health service in all humanitarian settings that involves multi-sectoral supports and requires its coordinated implementation—for example, through a cross-cluster or cross-sectoral working group. This coordination would enable quality assurance and accountability of aid agencies to their beneficiaries and would mean the consistency of the multidisciplinary ground values.

The Sphere Project Handbook identifies MH needs as the cross-cutting theme and an area of concern in disaster response, and addresses individual, group, or general vulnerability issues. Some of the greatest sources of vulnerability and suffering in disasters arise from the complex emotional, social, physical, and spiritual effects of disasters. Many of these reactions are normal and can be overcome with time. The Sphere underscores that is essential to organize locally appropriate MH and psychosocial supports that promote self-help, coping, and resilience among affected people. In each humanitarian sector, the manner in which aid is administered has a psychosocial impact that may either support or cause harm to affected people. Aid should be delivered in a compassionate manner that promotes dignity, enables self-efficacy through meaningful participation, respects the importance of religious and cultural practices, and strengthens the ability of the community to support holistic well-being. Humanitarian action is strengthened if at the earliest appropriate moment, affected people are engaged in guiding and implementing the disaster response (Sphere, 2014).

Yet, this exceptionally important initiative just scratched the surface of the problems scaffolded in humanitarianism by that time, and some NGOs, including Médecins Sans Frontières (MSF), criticized the project and its approach for "not taking enough risks" and for its disproportionate reliance on standards for technical interventions and not on the rights of affected populations. The position paper expressed concerns that this reliance would have reduced humanitarian response "to a simple mechanical and material exercise, devoid of its humanitarian ethos … or to business to be performed only according to technical standards" (SanJuan, 2003, p. 3). Despite of all the controversies, the Sphere Project has been a major step in establishing the coordination in humanitarian interventions and recognizing the key role of psychosocial supports in alleviating suffering.

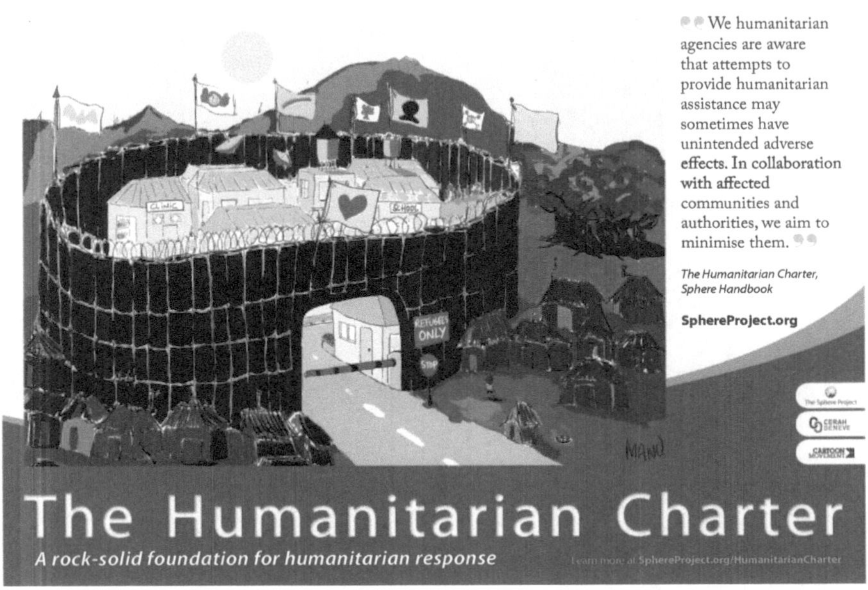

Figure 3.1 Aid Unintended Effects (By Manu. The SphereProject.org, used with permission)

I want to thank the Sphere Project for allowing me to use their cartoons and posters to illustrate the principles outlined in the Humanitarian Charter. These cartoons also provided me with the opportunity to hypothesize about the collateral problems arising when applying these principles.

The "Aid Unintended Effects" poster (Figure 3.1) demonstrates the unintended price for a humanitarian intervention and underscores that professional competencies must ethically accompany good intentions to reduce harm and minimize the potentially negative consequences for the affected populations.

The "Right to Life with Dignity" poster (Figure 3.2) appeals to NGOs where it emphasizes the importance of protecting dignity and respect of affected populations in aid delivery. In the situation shown on the poster, the NGO offers obviously humiliating clothes to the survivors. Which is never a good idea. At the same time, this picture spotlights the unexpected dilemma—what would be more important, dignity or lifesaving? What if the only available choices are not conducive to protecting dignity? Should NGOs deliver inappropriate clothes if these are the only clothes available or wait for a better opportunity? The humanitarian principle of accountability suggests the answer to this question includes delegating the decision-making power to survivors and letting them decide what's best for them.

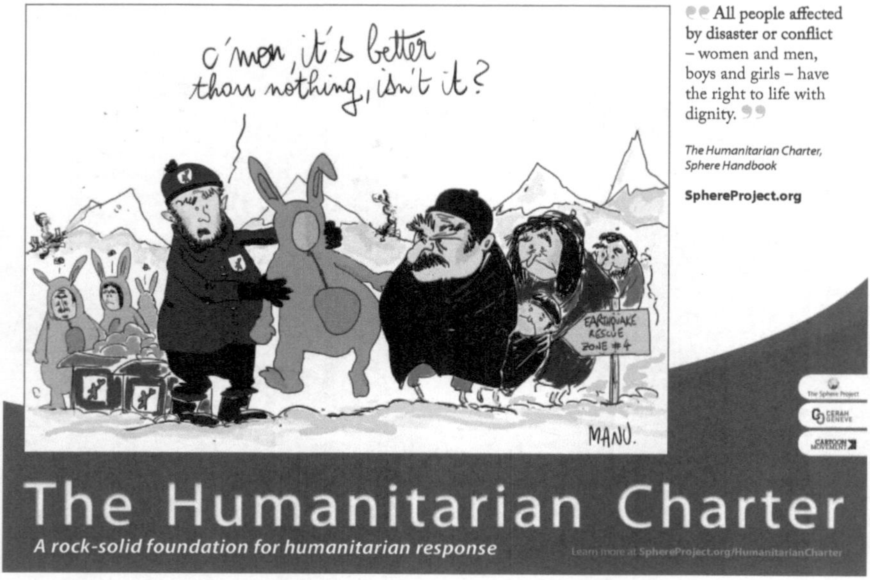

Figure 3.2 Life with Dignity (By Manu. The SphereProject.org, used with permission)

3.2 The NGO Code of Conduct

Code of conduct typically institutes the formal policies, procedures, and enforcement mechanisms that spell out the moral and ethical expectations of the organization. The NGO Code of Conduct has been a logical step in establishing standards for organizations involved in humanitarian work (Code of Conduct, 1994). It was conceived as a voluntary set of regulations enforced by the will of the organizations accepting it to maintain the standards it lays out. It has been adopted by nine of the largest humanitarian networks or agencies (see IFRC, 1994) and serves as a guide for international NGOs operating in the midst of violent conflicts, working to limit their harmful effects and maximize their contributions. This Code seeks to safeguard high standards of behavior while maintaining independence and effectiveness in disaster relief. It also defines and describes specific actions and practices to be encouraged or avoided for NGOs concerned about strengthening health systems in the countries where they work.

It is important to note that the Code of Conduct only applies to humanitarian actors and is not binding for organizations such as military forces or for-profit companies that may deliver assistance to communities affected by disaster. In the event of armed conflict, its clauses are to be interpreted and applied in conformity with international humanitarian law. This is also a reason why the principle of neutrality, which is directly related to the special international role of the Red Cross, is not included in the Code of Conduct.

The NGO Code of Conduct (Code of Conduct, 1994) has 10 articles that fall into two types: (1) Articles 1–4 are required, and (2) Articles 5–10 are aspirational yet important for quality humanitarian work:

1. The humanitarian imperative comes first.
2. Aid is given regardless of the race, creed, or nationality of the recipients and without adverse distinction of any kind. Aid priorities are calculated on the basis of need alone.
3. Aid will not be used to further a particular political or religious standpoint.
4. We shall endeavor not to be used as an instrument of government foreign policy.
5. We shall respect culture and custom.
6. We shall attempt to build disaster response on local capacities.
7. Ways shall be found to involve program beneficiaries in the management of relief aid.
8. Relief aid must strive to reduce vulnerabilities to future disaster as well as meeting basic needs.
9. We hold ourselves accountable to both those we seek to assist and those from whom we accept resources.
10. In our information, publicity, and advertising activities, we shall recognize disaster victims as dignified human beings, not hopeless objects.

The adoption of the Code of Conduct has affirmed the standards and ethical guidance for the humanitarian movement. However, many years after adopting the Code, its effectiveness is still being questioned. Hilhorst (2005, p. 364) outlined a number of limitations suggesting that "the code does not provide … clear pro-active regulation with respect to the provision of humanitarian aid." She did express the belief that the careful language makes the code comprehensive and appropriate as an instrument for discussing policy, although it also makes it less useful for NGOs seeking guidance for their actions and for purposes of accountability. At the same time, the voices of caution warned about the danger of overreliance on codes of conduct at the price of disparaging humanitarian values.

A recent example of the conflict between a code and the humanitarian values, or codes developed by establishments with different agenda, was the code of conduct for non-governmental organizations operating in the Mediterranean Sea drafted by Italian government looking to stem a flow of migrants into the country. According to data released by the interior ministry only in January–June 2017 some 85,217 migrants have come to Italy. Among the proposed new rules will be a ban on making phone calls or firing flares that might signal to human traffickers that they could push their migrant boats out to sea. The NGO vessels will also be obliged to let police travel with them to help root out any human traffickers hidden amongst the migrants. In addition, the boats will no longer be allowed to transfer refugees to other ships, but will instead have to bring them to port themselves, limiting their operations. Amnesty International and Human Rights Watch voiced concerns that the proposals could have a disastrous impact on NGO mission because it contradicts the point 4 of NGO code of conduct which states that humanitarians shall endeavor not to be used as an instrument of government foreign policy (Balmer, 2017).

3.3 Ethics of Global Mental Health

The Role of Professional Ethics

Professional ethics is a key component of professional and institutional identity. A code of ethics articulates basic values, sets the ideals, standards, and moral principles established by a profession and adopted by members as guidance for professional conduct and decision-making. Examples of professional organizations within the MH industry in the United States that have their own code of ethics include the American Psychological Association, the American Psychiatric Association, the National Association of Social Workers, and the American Counseling Association. The first code of ethics specifically for traumatologists was developed by Williams (2012) for the Association of Traumatic Stress Specialists (ATSS). The contents of these professional codes are not mutually contradicting and reflect the shared understanding of what it means to be an ethical health care professional.

The Need for a Broader Framework

The need for special ethics for GMH work is rooted in its unique mission and challenges. This work exposes professionals to complex moral choices and professional dilemmas where unethical practices tarnish the image of the profession, undermine the spirit of humanitarianism, and compromise the safety and well-being of both the providers and the people they serve.

Several researchers have noted limitations of the standards outlined by the professional associations, indicating the need for a broader frame of reference when working in the humanitarian context. One limitation relates to the positional statement of the American Psychological Association Ethics Code (APA, 2002), which states that the professional code is intended to provide guidance and standards of professional conduct to cover *most* situations encountered by psychologists. Cherepanov (2017a) demonstrated that GMH specialists often face *unprecedented* situations that require moving away from preconceived normative approaches toward establishing a frame of reference that is rooted in the humanitarian values and professional competencies of a provider.

Jenson (1997, p. 7), for instance, suggested that, in a disaster, the traditional tools of "objective" logic, rationality, and consistency may not be adequate, and the disaster management should be primarily governed by humanitarian values. Mackenzie, McDowell, and Pittaway (2007) and Pittaway, Bartolomei, and Hugman (2010, p. 13) echoed this, emphasizing the need in special ethical considerations to ensure the protection of participants when conducting humanitarian research, as well as the accuracy and relevance of the data. A study by Chuimento, Khan, Rahman, and Frith (2016) also demonstrated the limitations of the applicability of existing normative frameworks in relation to humanitarian research. They argued that ethical research conduct is not a product of adherence to a set of rules but of a mutually respectful encounter; they called for increased attention to documenting this process, building empirical evidence that critically considers the ethical difficulties in undertaking MH research in complex contexts and with complex populations.

De Torrente and Stobbaerts (2008) detailed similar considerations, pointing out the conceptual limitations of medical ethics in a humanitarian context. They examined the governing values of the humanitarian medical organizations, such as Doctors Without Borders (or MSF), and determined that medical ethics provide useful points of reference in highlighting instances where patients' interests should take precedence over policy or legislation. However, medical ethics do not constitute a clear guideline in humanitarian contexts. Not only are there different ethical approaches, but different ethical values often clash and require arbitration.

There are more specialized indications pointing out the limited applicability of the professional ethics in humanitarian contexts, as specifically referred to the medical ethics, globalization processes, and the humanitarian innovations. De Torrente and Stobbaerts (2008) believed that professional medical ethics are limited to only addressing health-related matters, whereas humanitarian catastrophes engulf people's entire lives. Benatar, Lister, and Thacker (2010, p. 143) proclaimed that in the current deteriorating economic and political climate a new balance of values and new ways of thinking and acting that transcend national and institutional boundaries are needed. Furthermore, Sheather et al. (2016) argued that the dynamic process of innovations may not fit with the conventional ethics framework, and any innovative projects may introduce additional risks for populations even if human participants are not directly involved. To resolve this dilemma, they suggested the use of high-level principles that have been developed for humanitarian innovation, although there is a lack of guidance for how these should be applied in practice. They proposed a Médecins Sans Frontières Ethics Framework for Humanitarian Innovation, and offered a self-guided decision-making algorithm for nonmedical innovators.

From Normative to Values-Based Ethics

Professional ethics establish personal, organizational, and corporate norms of conduct expected of professionals and set the rules for professional interactions. They are developed as a response to unethical practices, contain prescriptions about the course of action in morally ambiguous situations, and are concerned with what is the right and the wrong thing to do, or how one ought to act, morally speaking (Cavalier, 2014). Most are based on knowledge from ethical principles, legal precedents, and evidence-based medicine to draw solutions to ethical dilemmas (Goldenberg, 2005).

Value-based ethics, on the other hand, rely on a system of values that can be viewed, as Rokeach (1973) suggested, as broad preferences concerning the most appropriate courses of actions or outcomes. In GMH, where professionals work in unprecedented situations with no right or wrong solutions and ethical guidelines do not give clear directions or indicate which ethical imperative to follow, the values are left to guide decision-making. This approach has been finding growing support among MH and humanitarians professionals.

Behnke (2005) defined ethics as thinking about reasons in terms of values. He described the ethical practice of psychology as being mindful of the values that inform our clinical work, especially when those values compete with one another. This means that ethics help to navigate morally ambiguous situations and make difficult choices when none of the solutions are good—ethical guidance would not be needed if it were clear which choice was the right and moral one. Beauchamp and Bowie (1993) argued that in and of themselves, ethics codes are unlikely to influence individuals to be more ethical in the conduct of business. To be effective, ethics codes must be part of a value system that permeates the culture of the organization, and that, at a minimum, the code of conduct should be the subject of ethics training that focuses on actual dilemmas likely to be faced by members of the organization. Kohrt, Marienfeld, Panter-Brick, Tsai, and Wainberg (2016), for example, argued that the training programs in professional practice must incorporate the core values and competencies guiding the GMH work.

Table 3.1 compares the paradigms of normative frameworks reflected in professional codes and the proposed values-based framework for ethics of GMH.

Defining Ethics for GMH

To summarize, a need for special ethics in GMH is based on the following:

- Global MH professionals face unique professional and personal challenges when serving highly vulnerable populations in settings with complex needs and limited professional support.

Table 3.1 Professional Code of Ethics (Normative Ethics) and the Ethics of GMH (Values-Based Framework)

Normative Ethics (Professional Code of Ethics)	*Values-Based Ethics (Ethics for GMH)*
Contain profession-specific norms	Contain profession-specific AND multi-disciplinary humanitarian values
Based on precedents	Can be applied to unique and complex situations
Exerts absolute values	Emphasizes contextual relevance of values
Offers solutions	Offer the decision-making process
Rely on norms and prescriptions	Rely on professional competency
Non-negotiable, accepted as a whole	Allow prioritizing and negotiation

- A professional code of ethics is normative, based on precedents, and designed for typical situations, while in GMH the professionals often work in unique and unprecedented situations where they have to rely on their judgment, professional values, and competencies which call for a values-based frame of reference.
- In GMH, values-based ethical guidelines ensure accountability, flag unethical practices, and assist MH professionals with problem-solving in complex dilemmas.
- The high price for any ethical mistakes puts beneficiaries and aid workers at risk and can compromise the delivery of humanitarian aid.

In GMH work, the ethics serve to:

- set ground principles for professional interactions and decision-making;
- prioritize humanitarian values and accountability;
- establish a broader frame of reference in situations where professional values collide;
- guide planning and implementations of the interventions, or "how to do it right";
- flag unethical practices, or "what not to do";
- ensure safety, self-awareness, and self-care.

It is proposed that the ethics for GMH are defined as the system of professional and multidisciplinary values, competencies, and standards that provide guidance and frame of reference for reasoning the complex professional and moral dilemmas arising within the humanitarian context.

3.4 Developing an Ethical Framework

Identifying Governing Values

The Sphere Project affirmed the importance of the humanitarian standards in multidisciplinary humanitarian action. It affirmed the soundness of the presumption that when multidisciplinary providers operate, they must be able to rely on the shared values without compromising their professional standards. The path towards reconciling the multidisciplinary and professional agenda is not new: in the recent past, the development of the integrated primary care model accumulated experience of bringing together the multidisciplinary team members, forming a common agenda and making them agree on goals and outcome indicators while developing compatible assessments and protocols (Committee on the Future of Primary Care, 1996; DeGruy, 1996).

We will be using the Humanitarian Charter principles as a starting point in organizing the values governing GMH work into the values-based framework that would strengthen the GMH role as a dependable and trustworthy partner in

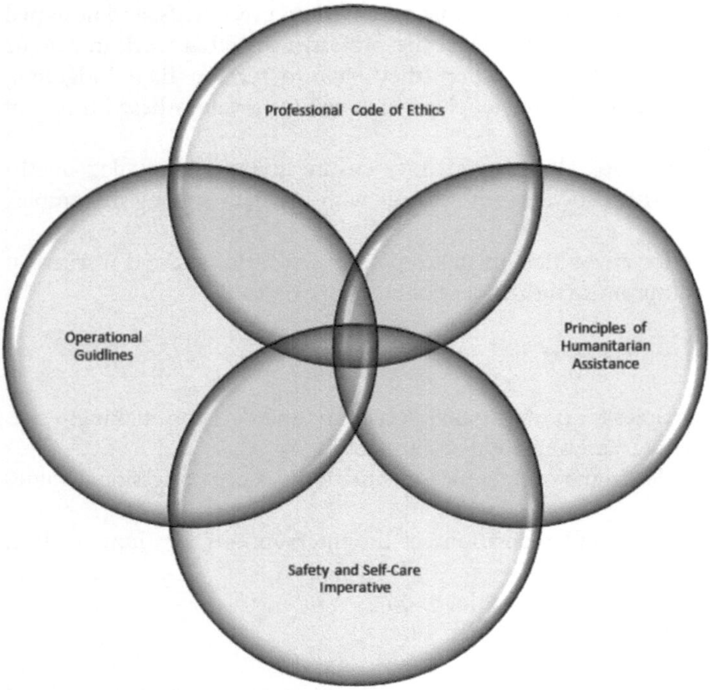

Figure 3.3 The System of Values Governing Global Mental Health

collaborative humanitarian action. In doing so, the first step would be to determine what these governing values are and what their interplay is when approaching ethical problems in GMH.

Because GMH plays such an important role in multidisciplinary collaborations, its work is influenced by different categories of values. They are safety and self-care, professional code of ethics, operational guidelines (IASC, 2007), and humanitarian principles (Cherepanov, 2017a). In Figure 3.3, the central overlapping area signifies the values governing the GMH practice.

Defining the Roles and Setting Up Priorities: Imperative, Normative, Prescriptive, or Aspirational Values

Once the values composing the ethical framework are determined, the next logical step is to examine their role and interrelation. It is possible to assume that different values can have different primacy and play different roles in decision-making, and that this role can be imperative, normative, prescriptive, or aspirational (Cherepanov, 2017a).

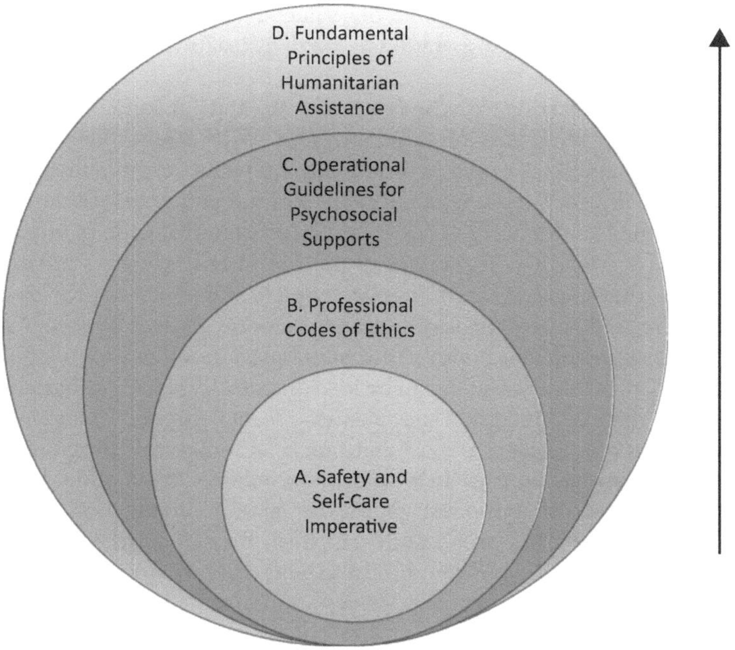

Figure 3.4 Interplay Between Multidisciplinary and Professional Values in Global Mental Health

- *Imperative values.* Safety and self-care.
  - Imperative values are nonnegotiable and carry absolute operational priority.
- *Normative values.* Professional code of ethics.
  - Normative values establish standards for professional conduct. In GMH, examples can be codes of ethics by the American Psychological Association, American Psychiatric Association, American Counseling Association, or National Association of Social Work (APA, NASW, ACA).
- *Prescriptive values.* Operational or strategic guidance.
  - Prescriptive values determine professional strategies that have been proven to be both effective and ethical.
- *Aspirational values.* Humanitarian principles.
  - Humanitarian principles reaffirm the humanitarian commitment and professional ideals and serve as a moral compass in professional decision-making.

Figure 3.4 establishes the interplay of values governing GMH, which is based on the role they play in professional decision-making. The values are presented as a set of concentric circles, and their position depends on whether they are normative, binding, prescriptive, or aspirational. The central placement of values reflects their precedence in decision-making, while the values placed on the periphery serve as aspirational or strategic (operational) guidance allowing for broader interpretations.

Let's look at these levels starting with the center and moving outward. Figure 3.4 points out the absolute priority and the imperativeness of the safety, followed by a professional code of ethics, strategic (operational) guidelines for psychosocial interventions, and finally, the fundamental principles of humanitarian assistance. The centrally positioned values of the A and B levels (professional code of ethics, safety and self-care) are binding. The values of the C and D levels are similarly important; however, they are aspirational and prescriptive and meant to provide a moral and operational guidance. Historically, these values themselves have been a work in progress reflecting the developments in humanitarian action.

Assigning the different roles to values can be instrumental in making programmatic decisions. For example, imagine a specialist who must design a MH support program for survivors of a disaster and wants to make sure that this program is aligned with the professional and multidisciplinary standards. What should the tactic be? For this, we check the proposal against the values in an outward direction starting from A (safety). If a proposal doesn't meet the standards on any of the levels, it needs to revert to the previous level and be revised. We start from core level A because safety of the aid workers is always an undisputed priority, and if safety is not assured, other programmatic concerns may not be as relevant. In our case, this can mean postponing launching the program until it is safer or changing its location. After risks are evaluated and there is confidence in reasonable safety, the next step would be to check whether the proposed interventions carry any potential for conflicting with standards outlined by the professional code of ethics. Next, we check if they are aligned with the operational guidelines for psychosocial interventions (see more in Chapter 7), and finally, whether they are consistent with the spirit of humanitarianism (see more in Chapter 6).

CHAPTER 4

Professional and Personal Challenges in Humanitarian Work

4.1 Humanitarian Crisis, Complex Emergency, and Post-Crisis Recovery

GMH interventions are carried out in the settings affected by the humanitarian crises, complex emergencies, or daily struggles of post-crisis recovery where the relief and recovery of a population is complicated by ongoing violence, broken infrastructure, and lack of resources. Regardless of the type of disaster, survivors are left in urgent of need of lifesaving assistance such as shelter, food, water, and health care. The categorization of a crisis is an important step in planning the humanitarian response, which determines the needs, the role of GMH, and the operational modalities of the interventions: see the explanation of the 5Rs operational modalities in Chapter 1. Figure 4.1 presents the classification of the humanitarian crises invoking the systemic vulnerabilities in the affected populations.

The Humanitarian Coalition (n.d) has defined a humanitarian crisis or humanitarian disaster as an event or series of events that presents a critical threat to the health, safety, security, or well-being of a community or other large group of people, usually over a wide area, and that can be characterized by the vulnerability of the affected population. "Vulnerability" refers to a reduced capacity of individuals or groups to resist and recover from life-threatening hazards and is most often connected to poverty. That is, poor populations are more likely to be more vulnerable to manmade or natural disasters because of the limited resources. Within affected communities, the most vulnerable groups typically include children, pregnant and nursing women, migrants, and displaced people.

According to the Humanitarian Coalition (n.d), a humanitarian emergency occurs when vulnerable populations are unable to withstand the negative consequences by themselves. Armed conflicts, epidemics, famine, natural disasters, and other major emergencies may all involve or lead to a humanitarian crisis that extends beyond the mandate or capacity of any single agency. Each humanitarian crisis is caused by different factors and equires a tailored response.

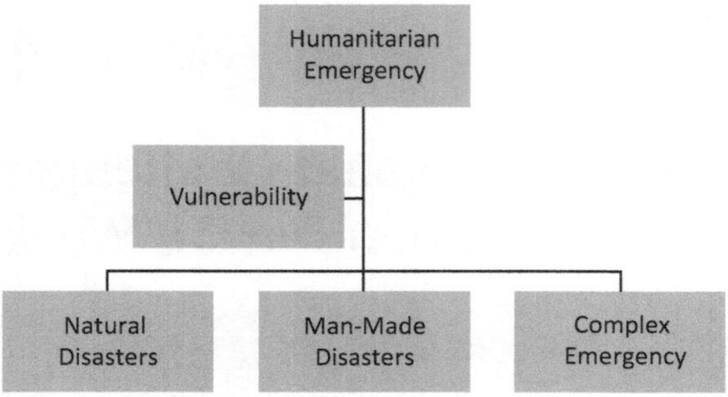

Figure 4.1 Classification of Humanitarian Emergencies (Humanitarian Coalition, http://humanitariancoalition.ca/what-is-a-humanitarian-emergency)

Complex Emergency

The Robert S. Strauss Center for International Security and Law (CCAPS, n.d) have stated the opinion that complex emergency situations are growing worldwide as conflicts become persistent and widespread, demographic patterns across the developing world change, income inequality deepens, and the poorest are subject to increased hazards due to climate change. The Center's position document has expressed belief that complex emergencies are responsible for cycles of conflict, high civilian mortality, a reversal of development goals, and perpetuating instabilities that are difficult to combat in post-conflict environments.

A complex emergency (CE) is a form of humanitarian crisis that occurs as a result of several factors or events that prevent a large group of people from accessing their fundamental needs, such as food, clean water, or safe shelter. The WHO views CEs as situations where a crisis has presented unique challenges due to its systemic impact, and defines CEs as

> situations of disrupted livelihoods and threats to life produced by warfare, civil disturbance, and large-scale movements of people, in which any emergency response has to be conducted in a difficult political and security environment. Complex emergencies combine internal conflict with large-scale displacements of people, mass famine or food shortage, and fragile or failing economic, political, and social institutions. Often, complex emergencies are also exacerbated by natural disasters.
>
> (Wisner & Adams, 2002)

To summarize, complex emergencies are characterized by:

- extensive violence and loss of life, massive displacements of people, widespread damage to societies and economies;
- the need for large-scale, multifaceted humanitarian assistance;

- the hindrance or prevention of humanitarian assistance by political and military constraints;
- significant security risks for humanitarian relief workers in some areas.

Population displacement, disruption of societal and community infrastructure, and mass trauma create a particular complexity of needs in affected populations. Cherepanov (2016) argued that a complex emergency destroys social and psychological infrastructure, compromises the recovery and perpetuates individual and collective trauma. A complex emergency hinders the community's ability to protect and support community members as it evokes a sense of hopelessness and helplessness and carries the potential to further demoralize, disempower the community, and overwhelm its capacity to cope. This contributes to further victimization and marginalization of vulnerable groups, and can have long-lasting political, social, economic, and psychological impacts (Cherepanov, 2011, 2015a, 2016).

Relief or Development

InterAction (2012) has recognized the importance of both relief and post-conflict recovery, and also transitioning from one state to another. The relief means attending to the immediate, pressing, and life-or-death needs of the affected population, while the recovery focuses on the long-term goals such as building capacity and resilience and sustainable economic and social developments. In a post-conflict setting, the population is often left without basic services and protection; they experience daily stresses of extreme and lingering poverty, community violence, and no access to health care for years beyond the initial emergency. Determination of whether it is more important to allocate resources to immediate relief or recovery efforts has become an extremely contentious issue, which came to the fore at the World Humanitarian Summit (see Chapter 2).

Holtzman (1999) traced the historical roots of this dilemma to aid groups becoming over focused on the immediate goal of saving lives and losing the bigger picture. With this in mind, he proposed reconciliation by suggesting that this "relief or development" dichotomy is artificial, as they are not separate endeavors but are actually sequential within a more comprehensive approach. While saving lives is always a priority, aiding societies engaged in and emerging from conflict helps to make transition more successful, leading to less violence and, at the end, saving more lives. Holtzman saw a solution to this conflict of agendas in forming partnerships between relief and development institutions early on in conflict situations, which would mean designing international aid to promote the social and economic reknitting of societies—a precondition for sustainable peace and the prevention of escalating violence.

Echoing this approach, Cherepanov (2016) believed that GMH should always be concerned about the sustainability of the recovery when responding to pressing humanitarian needs. It is proposed that the "relief or development" dilemma be replaced with a "transition from relief to development" strategy, with an understanding that the stronger recovery and development can reduce the need for emergency relief in the future and mitigate the transition to a more stable post-crisis setting.

4.2 Role of Global Mental Health Professionals in Settings with Complex Needs: IASC and CBPR Models

IASC Model: Mental Health and Psychosocial Supports in Emergencies

The complex and multilayered populational needs in an emergency require orchestrated intervention and supports from professionals and grassroots organizations, NGOs, the private and public sectors, service providers, researchers, and advocates. To tackle this ambitious task, the Interagency Standing Committee (IASC) issued guidelines (IASC, 2007) aimed at etsablishing a system of multi-layered complementary interventions that are organized according to different levels of MH needs. The role of GMH providers within the IASC framework will be further discussed using examples from the Last Mile Health project conducted in Liberia in the aftermath of the Côte d'Ivoire refugee crisis in 2011, when refugees fleeing sectarian violence overwhelmed the neighboring rural and impoverished regions of Liberia—a country recovering from 14 years of civil war (Cherepanov, 2016).

The IASC *Guidelines on Mental Health and Psychosocial Support in Emergeny Settings* (MHPSS) (IASC, 2007) is probably the most known and employed model in GMH. Paul, Sanson-Fisher, and Carey (2013) have attributed the success of the psychosocial approach to its holistic nature and its contribution to reconciliation of professional-driven and consumer-driven paradigms in MH. They expressed the hope that, in the future, any evaluation of its effectiveness wil be based not only on consumer satisfaction but also include research into its practice and professional assessment. The ground assumption of this well-organized model stems from the idea that in a complex emergency it is impossible to separate MH from social needs, and that the interventions must be tailored to survivors' needs (de Jong, 2011; de Jong & Kleber, 2001).

The Role of GMH Professionals According to the IASC Model

The IASC guidelines (2007, p. 9) view advocacy as a useful tool for promoting appropriate MH and psychosocial supports and in addressing gaps in recommended responses. The IASC model recommends interventions that are most appropriate at four different levels of MH needs so they may establish a complementary system of psychosocial supports in emergencies. The described levels of need are: basic services and security, community and family supports, focused non-specialized supports, and specialized services, and corresponding interventions are presented in the form of an intervention pyramid in Figure 4.2 (IASC, 2007, pp. 12–13).

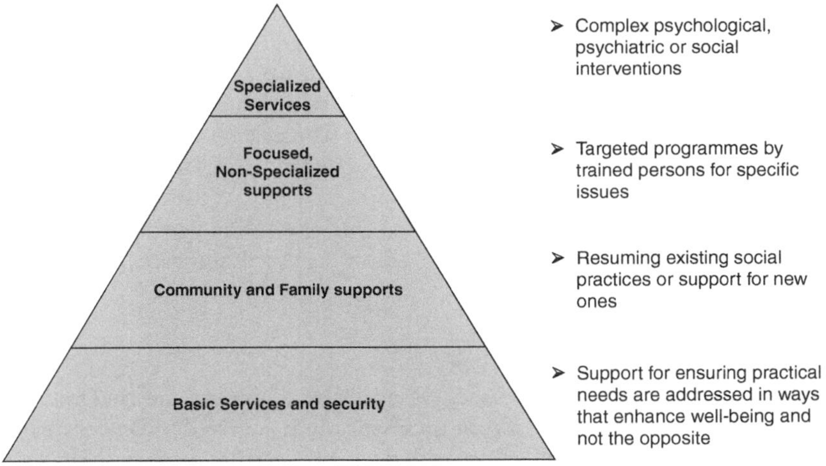

Figure 4.2 IASC Intervention Pyramid for Mental Health and Psychosocial Supports in Emergencies (IASC, 2007, pp. 12–13)

Next, we will discuss the needs-relevant role of GMH at and illustrate it with examples of intervention, starting from the bottom level (basic services and security) and working our way up to the top of the pyramid (specialized services).

Basic Services and Security

There are non-mental health NGOs that are responsible for food, water, shelter, and/or sanitation, and that specialize in delievering humanitarian aid. While the role of GMH professionals is limited at this level of basic needs, they can assist by advocating that aid be delivered in a culturally competent, trauma-informed manner to ensure the consumers' dignity, protection of vulnerable groups, and social justice.

> Such advocacy was needed in Liberia when the UNHCR delivered long-needed humanitarian aid to the remote region of Grand Gedeh county of Liberia. There, food was distributed to the refugee camps, but the families who hosted the refugees were not eligible for this aid. This perceived injustice caused discord and tension in the community, and increased hostility toward the refugees. The NGO's advocacy eventually helped to adjust the protocol.
>
> (E. Cherepanov, personal communication, June, 2011)

Community and Family Supports

The role of the MH professional changes when they support individuals who, though able to maintain their MH and psychosocial well-being, still need assistance in accessing key community and family supports. In a complex emergency, when there are significant disruptions in family and community networks due to displacement, family separation, community fears, and distrust, the IASC has recommended that responses include activation of social networks such as women's groups, youth clubs and initiatives, assisted mourning and communal healing ceremonies, mass communication on constructive coping methods, supportive parenting programs, educational activities, and family tracing and reunification.

The CBPR model that further defines the role of a GMH provider in mobilizing community supports is discussed below in the designated part of this chapter.

Focused Non-Specialized Supports

At the next level of MH needs, focused non-specialized supports are vital for individuals who have experienced severe traumatization, survived violence, or lost family members; are having difficulties with sleep, hypervigilance, angry outbursts, social isolation, and stress-related health problems; but who have generally been able to manage their lives and attend to their daily needs. These individuals may need focused counseling and/or individual, family, or group supports supervised by MH professionals.

In Liberia, like in many other places in the world, trauma survivors rarely reach out for help, and most trauma-related referrals come from concerned family members, primary care providers, outreach workers, and peers. According to Green et al. (2003), MH services often carry a stigma, and participation in a standalone MH program can expose survivors by simply seeking treatment. Medical services are perceived to be a more socially acceptable alternative, which is one reason why GMH has geared toward the implementation of integrated models that can assure continuity of care and successful referrals between primary care and behavioral health programs.

> Many trauma survivors have concurrent medical conditions that primary care providers identify and make referrals for. For example, psychosomatic complaints (headaches, stomachaches, ambiguous medical conditions) are often the initial reason for seeking treatment. Other requests for services come from survivors' families who are concerned for a family member whose behavior changed, becoming jumpy, angry, lazy, isolated, neglectful, or depressed. Observations of insomnia, overreacting, emotional outbursts, self-medicating with alcohol, and "thinking too much" (i.e. anxiety) were also common complaints from family members seeking assistance for a loved one.
>
> (E. Cherepanov, personal communication, June 20, 2011)

Specialized Services

The top layer of the IASC pyramid represents the small percentage of populations that require specialized services and treatment. These are individuals with serious mental illness and/or debilitating trauma who have experienced significant difficulties in basic daily functioning. Specialized services including treatment, risk and crisis management, and counseling provided by professional MH specialists with expertise in trauma, mental disorders, and mental illness. Training the national MH specialists plays an important role in building the referral system and training other providers. Dr. Janice Cooper who has been training MH specialists in Liberia said

> I didn't dare dream in 2010 when I came home after years in the US that in 2017 we would have trained 232 MH clinicians, scores of mid-levels in mhGAP, have trained 64 clinicians with specialty in children and have 6 school-based health centers.
>
> (E. Cherepanov, personal communication, December 1, 2017)

> As the the Last Mile-Health project demonstrated in 2012, in rural Liberia, specialized services have presented particular challenges in the absence of specialists, medications, and referral systems. The only psychiatric hospital in Liberia's capital, Monrovia, was hardly accessible due to lack of transportation and unnavigable roads during the rainy season. This community usually recognized and demonstrated concern toward individuals with serious impairment and actively advocated for their access to treatment.
>
> (E. Cherepanov, personal communication, May 30, 2012)

As I often observed, even in countries such as Liberia, where people are generally kind to those suffering from serious mental disorders or mental illnesses, having MH issues is still considered shameful. Similar to those held by many other cultures around the world, a widespread and very pervasive belief exists that mental illness is a punishment for sin or is caused by a curse. This stigmatizing belief has been particularly difficult to challenge. As one of the health care providers in training told me: "After your training, I now understand that mental illness is not contagious or caused by a curse, but I know one family where this was the case for sure!" (E. Cherepanov, personal communication, June 10, 2012). Limited availability of treatment opportunities can create morally difficult choices for providers and families. Most indigenous healing practices include prayer and the use of herbal remedies; whole others encompass the infliction of pain and humiliation, such as ritualistic beating (E. Cherepanov, personal communication, June 15, 2012). On the other hand, some traditional practices, which have been traditionally condemned as abusive by the professional community, may have been developed as harm reduction in the absence of better alternatives. For example, in some villages, residents use physical restraints on individuals with psychotic symptoms for their safety in the absence of anti-psychotic medications to physically prevent them from wandering away or potentially being assaulted or killed. Instead of just condeming these practices, the role of the MH professional in these situations can be to offer viable and safe alternatives through their work, such as teaching families and survivors about symptoms management.

Many things have improved in Liberia since then, which include training of several cohorts of MH providers by the Carter Center. At the time though, health care workers have shared frustration because they cannot ensure continuity of their care. In addition, the supply of psychotropic medications in remote areas is inconsistent. Even when medications become available, they are used with caution due to concerns about the likelihood of discontinuation (E. Cherepanov, personal communication, June 1, 2012). In this difficult situation, the most helpful intervention was found to be psychoeducation aimed at combating stigma and prejudice, training primary health workers and acompaniers, educating the family on how to support an individual with uncontrolled symptoms of mental illness, and health care advocacy.

CBPR Model: Community-Based Psychological Recovery in Complex Emergencies

The National Consensus Statement on Mental Health Recovery, SAMHSA (2004) defined MH recovery as the process of change through which individuals strive to improve their health and well-being, live a self-directed life, and strive to achieve their full potential. The community-based psychological recovery (CBPR) in a complex emergency model (Cherepanov, 2015a, 2016), emphasized the role of community in recovery, and operationalized strategies that enable MH professionals to mobilize and strengthen the community to facilitate and support psychological recovery. This model, the elements of which have been piloted in Chechnya, Chernobyl, Kosovo, Liberia, and Ukraine, is a strength-based approach aimed at mobilizing and strengthening recovery resources, improving access to supports, and sensitizing communities to the needs of vulnerable groups (Cherepanov, 2011, 2016).

The CBPR model is based on the assumption that the quality of community supports shapes psychological recovery in complex emergencies by providing a secure sense of self, supportive relationships, empowerment, social inclusion, and meaning. This assumption was based on Goodman et al.'s (1998) understanding of community as having a powerful protective influence that can mitigate social ills. Goodman et al. (1998, p. 840) also outlined the aspects that are key to this construct, including participation and leadership skills, informational and logistic resources, social networks, a sense of community, and an understanding of community history, community power, community values, and critical reflection.

The CBPR model links the community's recovery to the quality of community supports and the ability of survivors to acces them (Cherepanov, 2015a). According to this model, the mobilization of community-based protective factors, such as traditional mutual supports and conflict-resolution protocols, can be decisive elements for community engagement in the healing process. However, it is important that the suggested supports are built on and congruent to local cultural practice. For instance, the tradition of sharing one's positive and negative experiences in a group setting exists in many cultures—in countries of West Africa, for one, this is called the "Palava" tradition. In other cultures, such as the Northern Caucasus, the ritual of conversing while drinking coffee serves a similar purpose (E. Cherepanov, personal communication, April, 2016).

As stated earlier, community supports are vital for the individuals who have experienced severe traumatization, or lost family members, and are having difficulties with sleep, hypervigilance, angry outbursts, social isolation, and stress-related health problems, but who have generally been able to manage their lives and attend to their daily needs.

Unfortunately, complex emergencies destabilize or destroy the fabric of a community's social life and psychological supports. They overwhelm community resilience, undermine coping capacities, and heighten systemic vulnerabilities that have wider implications for the perpetuation of traumatization in the future. In the CBPR model, MH providers partner with the community to recognize and build upon community strengths and improve survivors' access to health care. This includes identification, mobilization, or restoration of community supports and destigmatization of MH issues. Training local MH providers and trauma workers, who are often survivors themselves, is crucial for the community self-reliance and sustainability of recovery.

4.3 External, Professional, and Personal Challenges

When working in complex emergencies, MH providers encounter exceptional challenges. Often, they work in volatile and unsafe environments where they have to make quick and effective decisions under duress in situations with high moral ambiguity, which emphasizes the need for guidance to support decision-making. The external, professional, and personal challenges listed below have been taken from the Sphere Project (2004), with some additional suggestions by aid workers in my training and workshops. The external and personal challenges are shared by GMH professionals as well as other humanitarian workers, and professional challenges are more specific to GMH work.

External Challenges

External challenges refer to the political, social, and logistic context of GMH work that MH professionals have little control over, yet which have a huge impact on aid delivery, MH interventions, and providers' well-being. Below are the external challenges identified by the Sphere Project (2004).

- security;
- politics;
- funding;
- logistics;
- rules, regulations, and values of the deploying organizations.

The strategies for reconciling the arising professional and moral values will be examined in Chapter 8.

Personal Challenges

Personal challenges can take a psychological toll on humanitarian workers, affect their psychological well-being and health, compromise safety, and lead to burnout. They include:

- physical and moral hardship;
- threats to personal safety;
- health-related risks;
- exposure to mass trauma and severe suffering;
- being separated from personal supports;
- facing moral ambiguities.

Professional Challenges

Professional challenges reflect the underlying conflict between the professional mission on one hand and the limited skills, tools, and resources on the other. For example:

- working with severe trauma and suffering;
- facing unique moral and professional dilemmas;
- compromised or nonexistent referral or continuity of care systems;
- limited access to professional supports and supervision;
- language barriers and working with interpreters affecting the quality of communication;
- serving populations from different cultures, where cultural differences are based on profoundly different lifestyles and accumulated trans-generational experiences (Cherepanov, 2015b);
- being part of a multidisciplinary and multicultural team—when focusing on the multicultural populations of people we serve, we tend to underestimate the cultural differences between providers who come from different countries. A professional culture also plays an important role: public health providers, psychologists, social workers, and psychiatrists may view a problem from different perspectives.

4.4 Exercise: Check Your Knowledge

This exercise aims to check the understanding of the material that is offered in this chapter.

1. Define humanitarian crisis.
2. Define complex emergency. Give recent examples.

3. Complex emergencies mostly occur in low-income countries. Can they happen in developed countries?
4. Did Hurricane Katrina in the United States qualify as a complex emergency? Explain your reasoning. What about Hurricaine Harvey?
5. How does declaring a complex emergency affect MH intervention strategies? (Use the CNN fast facts for this analysis: www.cnn.com/2013/08/23/us/hurricane-katrina-statistics-fast-facts/)
6. Name four levels of populational needs in the IASC model of MH and psychosocial interventions and supports.
7. Name two professional, two external, and two personal challenges in GMH.

CHAPTER 5

Managing Ethical Challenges in Global Mental Health

5.1 Humanitarian Research. Children as Research Subjects

GMH professionals work in various capacities and these different facets of the work come with specific ethical challenges, which will be discussed in this chapter.

Humanitarian Research as a Priority in GMH

> The ethical challenge is for researchers to add value to the lives of the people they are researching, recognizing them as subjects in the process and not simply as sources of data.
>
> (Pittaway et al., 2010, p. 231)

In 2014, the IASC declared humanitarian research a priority in mental health and psychosocial support (MHPSS), where it was recognized as a powerful tool for social justice, determination of needs, evaluating the impact of humanitarian assistance, planning and coordinating relief efforts, and the allocation of aid. Lambert (2015) further asserted that research in GMH enhances our understanding of the diversity of human resilience and the response to extreme stress and trauma and is used for advancing psychosocial interventions, innovations, and advocacy.

IASC defined research in GMH as:

> The systematic collection and analysis of data that applies to qualitative or ethnographic data (that can be observed) or quantitative data (that can be measured). This includes needs assessments; psychiatric epidemiology (study of distribution and cause of mental illness); monitoring and evaluation (M&E), social sciences research; as well as data collected for advocacy purposes.
>
> (IASC, 2014)

The IASC (2014) outlined their strategic agenda in addressing ethical challenges in GMH research:

- Ensure MHPSS research in emergencies benefits affected people.
- Design research to fill knowledge gaps in MHPSS theory and practice in emergencies.
- Avoid bad practice, such as research without satisfactory consent of participants.
- Better understand how to manage ethical challenges in MHPSS research during emergencies.

High Price for Overlooked Ethics

The importance of data for planning aid and the vulnerability of the research subjects elevate the role of ethical standards. At the same time, the ethical conduct of international researchers employing questionable research protocols has been brought to question (Loff & Black, 2000; Marshall & Batten, 2004; Pittaway et al., 2010; Shalala, 2000). Additionally, Ponterotto and Casas (1991) unveiled widespread issues such as exploitation of the ethnic and minority participants, negative impact on the community, and unreliable findings. "Fly in and fly out," "disaster tourism," disrespect to the local culture, disregard for the safety of participants and the future of the community, practices bordering on coercion, and avoiding addressing the validity of data, all undermine the integrity of humanitarian research and the usefulness of any collected data. It also erodes the community trust in researchers and impedes the image of humanitarianism. I have personally observed this troubling discourse and many aid workers have shared similar stories.

The Australian humanitarian Pittaway (Pittaway et al., 2010) declared that ethical regulations have been long overdue in field research and offered a disturbing glimpse into the state of affairs on the ground. Pittaway referred to her proposal to conduct a study with the women she was working with on the preparation of advocacy materials for the UN Commission on the Status of Women, various UN World Conferences, and the (then known as) Human Rights Commission. She knew of participants' need for change, their desire to tell their stories, and to advocate at the UN. The trusting relationship she had established allowed her to hear the true voice of participants.

The initial reaction of the women to the news that the research would be funded was disappointment—someone they had trusted as a trainer was now suggesting that they work with her as research subjects. Although the women had expressed the desire to have their stories told and their issues addressed at an international level, their deep fear of exploitation by researchers made them wary of participating in such a study. Their concerns were centered on the following (Pittaway et al., 2010, pp. 235–236):

- exploitation by previous researchers and journalists, including unauthorized publication of names and photos, leading at times to situations of danger for those participating in the research;

- false expectations of assistance from researchers;
- lack of feedback from research, including promised reports and photos, after giving time for interviews and disclosing personal stories;
- fear of backlash from government authorities and military leaders within camps;
- mistrust of white researchers by local workers and researchers;
- distrust of research done by researchers who "fly in and fly out" of camps and conflict zones without considering the local social, economic, and political consequences;
- lack of consultation about recommendations and strategies;
- the inability of many researchers to cope with the absolute horror of the experiences of research participants.

Ethical Challenges in Humanitarian Research

Marshall and Batten (2004) argued that the research relationship is one of a co-constructed nature and should not be determined by the boundaries of current ethical research and design practices. They went on to suggest that the ethics of contemporary academic research practices should be constantly evolving, and, despite theoretical limitations, should seek to break from "traditional-colonial theorizing about cross-cultural samples." Marshall and Batten (2004) concluded that conducting research across any cultural context requires intense attention to ethics, in large part because a cross-cultural research relationship inherently involves a dynamic of power. As members of colonial cultures, researchers have traditionally held power in the forms of money, knowledge, and "expertise" over their human subjects. Cascading from this foundation of power, the research relationship spawns other ethical issues of informed consent, control, research design, and data ownership.

The movement toward humanitarian accountability, professionalization, and quality management has placed humanitarian research at the top of humanitarian priorities in areas like patient safety research (WHO, 2013) and GMH research (Cherepanov, 2017b; Chiumento et al., 2016; Lambert, 2015). Multidisciplinary publications have affirmed the standards for conducting research outlined by the relevant professional associations and also highlighted the need for unique ethical considerations to ensure the protection of participants as well as the accuracy and relevance of data (Curry, Waldman, & Caplan, 2014; Mackenzie et al., 2007; Pittaway et al., 2010).

Chiumento et al. (2016) argued that ethical research conduct is not a product of adherence to a set of rules but of mutually respectful encounters and the documentation of this process, and of building empirical evidence for ethics in GMH research. The study expressed optimism that global initiatives can contribute to the development of an approach to applied ethics that responds appropriately to the specific issues raised in practice and that promotes ethical standards to

Table 5.1 Ethical Challenges in Humanitarian and Global Mental Health Research

Ethical Challenges	*Concerns*
Validity	Questionable cross-cultural validity of assessment tools Pathologizing suffering in Western approaches Difficulties translating Western terminology into the local language
Confidentiality	Breaches in confidentiality on sensitive issues such as sexual assault history, political affiliation, religious belief, and sexual orientation could put participants and their families in serious danger
Cultural appropriateness of the research protocols	Western ethnocentric thinking is characterized by universalized conceptualizations and informs academic research norms
Informed consent	The power differential between researchers and participants may lead to coercion in the data collection process, particularly when Westerners are working in low-resource areas Obtaining informed consent adds complexity when potential participants live in oppressive contexts or settings where they fear repercussions for declining participation
Sampling	Recruiting a truly representative sample
Emotional distress	Some inquiries in MH research have potential to invoke emotional distress, which may become problematic in the absence of a referral infrastructure
Duty to intervene or report	Raises questions about the ethical obligation in cases of information signaling imminent danger or harm
Data ownership	Who owns the researcher data: research body, participants, or community, and how should these data be communicated?

underpin research in emergencies. Lambert's (2015) literature review identified validity, confidentiality, informed consent, and cross-cultural relevance as areas of primary ethical concern in GMH. These areas and the relevant concerns are synthesized in Table 5.1.

Validity

When data are used to make important decisions concerning resource allocation, aid delivery, program development, or psychological interventions, it is important to ensure that the accuracy and relevancy of the needs assessment (Beyrer & Kass, 2002). While there were studies where researchers have been successfully working toward establishing validity of cultural idioms of distress (Bolton, 2001a, 2001b), the cultural congruency of Western concepts of mental disorders continued igniting concerns about pathologizing suffering, iatrogenesis, and the misuse of medication.

Lambert (2015) supported Wessells' (2009) point about how the difficulties of translating Western terminology into local languages can lead to misunderstandings and erroneous conclusions. Even though most of the globally used assessments at some point were validated and standardized for use with multicultural populations, an absolute language and cultural congruence is hardly attainable. The reasonable efforts to ensure the accuracy of translation may still not be enough to achieve true equivalence of meaning, as the questions or statements may carry different connotations for participants from different age groups, different villages, tribes, or stratums within the same culture or region.

To address these challenges, Prince (2008) suggested that to be valid, assessments across culture requires qualitative research to investigate the cultural relevance of the construct, then a careful translation and adaptation of a common measure, followed by pretesting and cognitive interviews on the populations to be tested. Bhutta (2004) and Allden et al. (2009) went on to argue that these risks to validity can be mitigated by careful planning and knowledge of local concerns and cultural norms, and by more widely employing the participatory action research (PAR) standards in humanitarian data collection. Within a PAR process, "communities of inquiry and action evolve and address questions and issues that are significant for those who participate as co-researchers" (Reason & Bradbury, 2008).

Confidentiality

In settings where community members are closely monitored, it may be impossible to guarantee that an individual's participation is confidential. In a politically volatile situation, participation in research in and of itself could compromise the safety of participants and breaches in confidentiality on sensitive issues such as sexual assault history, political affiliation, religious belief, and sexual orientation could put participants and their families in danger (Beyrer & Kass, 2002; Mackenzie et al., 2007; Pittaway et al., 2010).

Informed Consent

Voluntary and informed consent is the cornerstone of any ethical research. Leaning (2001) warned against ignoring the power differential between researchers and participants, particularly when Westerners are working in low- and low-middle-income countries (LLMIC) where any real or perceived coercion may easily affect the consent, the sampling, and the integrity of data. In such situations, the participants may feel that they have to participate "to please the researchers" or that their well-being or that of their family or community depends on their answers. Obtaining informed consent adds complexity when potential participants may fear repercussions either for declining to take part or consenting to participation (Allden et al., 2009; Chiumento et al., 2016; Ellis, 2007; Pittaway et al., 2010):

> When I go into a horrendous camp situation as a white researcher, the people are so desperate for any form of assistance they would agree to anything just on the off-chance that I might be able to assist. It makes asking for permission to interview them or take photographs a farce ... What does "informed consent" mean in an isolated refugee camp with security problems and no proper interpreters?
>
> (L. Bartolomei, personal communication, 2004, cited in Pittaway et al., 2010, p. 234)

Cultural Appropriateness of the Research Protocols

Rabionet, Santiago, and Zorilla (2009) argued that culturally competent research takes into account the diversity of the population when developing research ideas, conducting research, and exploring applicability of research findings. The researcher's cultural competencies are critical to ensure: (1) effective communication and interaction between researchers and study participants; (2) adequate analysis and interpretation of results as they relate to the patients/population; (3) appropriate engagement in study design and implementation for community-/population-based research that takes into account the diversity of the population when developing research ideas, conducting research, and exploring applicability of research findings.

Instructions, formulations of questions, and communication of the results are all culturally sensitive and could have different meaning in different cultures. For example, in some cultures certain instructions and questions may be perceived as intrusive or inappropriate. As Singer (1993) contends, the ethical consideration is a component of any human interaction, and the need for it increases when a relationship occurs across cultures, where conceptions of ethics can differ greatly. Singer saw the solution in a community-based partnership in developing research protocols that incorporate an ongoing process of communication and offer an ethical solution that is mutually beneficial to both researchers and cultural group members.

Sampling

Rabionet et al., (2009) proposed that cultural competence could help to improve participation of minority populations in studies, ensuring that different subgroups in the population are represented proportionally in research studies. At the same time, recruiting a truly representative sample in a setting with an oppressive regime can be problematic because of the limited access to the persecuted group and assuring safety for the participants. It also raises question about the degree to which a researcher can or should remain neutral when learning about ongoing human rights abuses (Beyrer & Kass, 2002; Ellis, 2007; Pittaway et al., 2010).

Data Ownership

Data ownership problems have become increasingly articulated as a major concern for research ethics, particularly when participants are recruited from marginalized groups. Darou, Kurtness, and Hum (1993) suggested that some ethical problems could be avoided by sharing data results and ownership with participants. Crittenden (2016) went on to suggest that, in the age of "big data," outside organizations should consider the ethics of data collection, analysis, and circulation. Unless the local populations have access to and some means to use it themselves, data can become another "extractive resource." Cherepanov (2017b) believes that there seems to be a reasonable expectation for a GMH researcher to develop recommendations on addressing the identified problems, and plan on reporting findings back to the community. A community that realizes how the research is beneficial for them would likely not feel exploited and would be more open to participate in research in the future.

Children as Research Subjects

The Grand Challenges in GMH initiative emphasized that children require particular attention for prevention and care (Collins et al., 2011). In humanitarian emergencies, children are the most vulnerable group, which means that humanitarian research with child participants must be held to the highest ethical standards. Next, we will review special provisions related to using children as research subjects within the areas of ethical concerns that have been previously identified (Cherepanov, 2017b).

Validity

The issue of validation of assessment tools for children from different cultures and contexts is even more pronounced than it is for adults because traditionally there have been fewer assessment tools for children to begin with. Cross-cultural variations in the expression of mental disorders can be even greater when considering developmental and gender factors. For instance, in my experience, teenage boys often adamantly deny the questioner statement "I cry too much," because affirmation could be perceived by others as a gender-incongruent "weakness." I also have concerns about the widespread belief I have encountered that, in the absence of standardized tools, it is acceptable to use proxy or similar instruments without checking their suitability and appropriateness.

Confidentiality

A breach in confidentiality on sensitive issues, such as child abuse, neglect, or maltreatment, can put children at risk. Children are often closely monitored by parents and the community and it can be difficult to ensure the privacy of their responses. I observed on many occasions how parents exert control over their children and do not allow them to meet with the provider in privacy. If they do, they expect children to report on everything that happened. Participation in the research by itself can expose children and compromise their safety, as parents or teachers may use their authority to put pressure on children to "tell the truth" about their responses. In addition, the published data, even when the individual identities are hidden, may still lead to blaming children for exposing the community in a negative light. This opens up a dilemma: how can we advocate for elimination of child abuse if children are put at risk for exposing this abuse? Gathering indirect and collateral data may be a safer approach in these situations.

To reduce risks for children, it is important that parents and community leaders participate in planning the research, and understand its goals as well as the non-disclosure agreement. It is crucial that all possible precautions be taken to ensure privacy of the records and that there be provisions for preserving the privacy of data in case of evacuation.

Informed Consent

The concerns about covert coercion in recruiting participants when people are in dire need are exponentially amplified when recruiting children who depend on their parents or other adults. Participatory action research can help to address any power differential between researchers and participants (Chiumento et al., 2016; Pittaway et al., 2010), which includes educating children and parents on how this research will be conducted, helping the community, and informing them that they can decline participation at any time without any repercussions or the need to return any offered reward or incentive.

Emotional Distress

The commonly used assessment tools often inquire about personal adverse experiences; this has the potential to cause emotional distress. Although Labott, Johnson, Fendrick, and Feeny (2013) argued that this happens in a very small percentage of the population with no reported adverse effects, their study was conducted on adults and may or may not be applicable to child populations. The WHO (2013) suggested that, as a result of their participation, research participants can become emotionally distressed, fearful, or anxious, and so WHO issued a special guidance on mitigating potential psychological risks for participants. It states that providers should anticipate any distress participants may experience as a consequence of the conduct of the study and be prepared to offer solutions (WHO, 2013, p. 15). Another example is the most recent clinical guidelines on "Responding to Children and Adolescents Who Have Been Sexually Abused," which were published while I was writing this book (WHO, 2017). The guidelines outline the strategies of helping frontline health workers, primarily from low-resource settings, in providing evidence-based, quality, trauma-informed care to survivors. The guidelines emphasize the importance of promoting safety, offering choices, and respecting the wishes and autonomy of children and adolescents.

Duty to Intervene

Using children as research subjects in GMH raises questions about the researcher's responsibility in the case of responses that suggest a child may be in imminent danger or that there is ongoing child abuse, neglect, or maltreatment. The WHO (2017) proposed a guideline stating that researchers, designated authorities, and health care providers should inform the child or adolescent and their non-offending caregivers about their obligation to report abuse and the limits of confidentiality before interviewing them. In reality, however, the implementation of this guideline may turn out to be a complicated task. There may not be any non-offending family members, and there is no guarantee that this information will not be shared. Furthermore, there may not be any available child protection agencies, and the authorities will not necessarily prioritize the children's safety.

Another related concern relates to establishing proper channels and methods of communication for the safety of children and the community if the revealed information indicates imminent danger. And what if this danger is not imminent but delayed? Who shall these finding be communicated to. Finding answers to these and similar concerns must be a part of thorough pre-planning.

Recommendations for Minimizing Ethical Risks in GMH Research: Ethical Review Boards

In the light of mounting criticism of integrity of humanitarian research, Leaning (2001) formulated stern recommendations for research in refugee and internally displaced populations that some have perceived as excessively stringent. Leaning (2001) argued that ethical researchers do the following:

- Undertake only those studies that are urgent and vital to the health and welfare of the study population.
- Restrict studies to those questions that cannot be addressed in any other context.
- Restrict studies to those that would provide important direct benefit to the individuals recruited to the study or to the population from which the individuals come.
- Ensure the study design imposes the absolute minimum of additional risk.
- Select study participants based on scientific principles without bias introduced by issues of accessibility, cost, or malleability.
- Establish highest standards for obtaining informed consent from all individual study participants, and where necessary and culturally appropriate, from heads of household and community leaders (but this consent cannot substitute for individual consent).
- Institute procedures to assess for, minimize, and monitor the risks to safety and confidentiality for individual subjects and their communities, now and for their future.
- Promote the well-being, dignity, and autonomy of all study participants in all phases of the research study.

The humanitarian community saw a powerful tool for humanitarian research in instituting the Ethical Review Boards (ERBs) to rigorously manage ethical challenges that may not be captured by research ethics guidelines. ERBs ensure oversight of the ethicality of the research and safeguard against unethical practices. According to Schopper et al. (2009), ethical reviews in humanitarian research are set to protect the dignity, rights, well-being, and welfare of research participants and communities and would act as an advocacy group for raising ethical awareness among scientists and humanitarian agencies that design and implement medical research in refugee settings. For example, Schopper et al. (2009) asserted the MSF-ERB's role in examining research protocols to make sure that the research is scientifically sound, pertinent, relevant, and beneficial for the community and/or the intended participants; that the methods by which the research will be conducted are rigorously validated; and that the participants' rights are respected and protected. The recommendations for the ERBs outline principles for ethical decision-making. The ground values for MSF-ERB operations include:

- *Collaborative partnership*. Researchers should engage in partnership with national and/or international research institutions as relevant and appropriate.
- *Community engagement*. Researchers should respect the community's values, culture, traditions, and social practices; involve the community in the design and implementation of research through a consultative process; and fairly share any financial and other rewards of the research.
- *Social value*. Beneficiaries should be clearly specified, and the importance of the health problems being investigated and the prospect of value of the research for the beneficiaries made clear.
- Efforts should be made *to avoid diverting resources* from health services for the conduct of research.
- *Scientific validity research design* should optimize possibilities of achieving the social value requirements. Research should be feasible given the social, political, and cultural environment and contribute to sustainable improvements in the local health care and physical infrastructure.
- *Fair selection of participants*. The study population should be selected in such a way as to ensure scientific validity of the research and minimize the risks of the research.
- *Favorable harm–benefit ratio protocols* should clearly assess potential harms and benefits to the study participants and the harm–benefit ratio for the community. The study community should be involved in establishing appropriate recruitment procedures and incentives for the participants. Consent procedures should be acceptable and practical within the study community.

In addition to the strategic directions on managing ethical challenges in GMH research described above, I suggest additional practical considerations that stem from my experience:

1. The local staff on the ground, community members, and peers can be instrumental and should be consulted in deciding the cultural appropriateness of the research protocols, instructions, and samples.
2. The researchers should partner with the community in developing culturally grounded research protocols.
3. In addition to individual consents, the participating community and especially the community leaders shall be informed about the research goals and how the data will be collected and used.
4. It is important that the results be reported back to the community so it can benefit from the findings. This establishes trust, which is vital for future collaboration, and helps to prevent the community from feeling exploited.
5. Extra efforts must be made to ensure the confidentiality of the responses and to keep the records and health-related information protected in case researchers have to evacuate.
6. The decision whether to participate as a research subject should not be linked to coercive practices such as receiving a substantive award. If a reward for participation is offered, the participant must be able to withdraw from participation without returning the award.
7. It is important that the interviewers be trained in psychological first aid and able to offer emotional support and appropriate referrals, if needed.

5.2 Trauma Work: Professional and Personal Boundaries

Williams (2010, 2012) saw the biggest challenge for traumatologists in moral ambiguities and the erosion of professional and personal boundaries where the ethical principles help to make trauma practitioners serve their clientele appropriately within a relationship of power inequity. Braak (2002) believed that diminished trauma survivor trust to the world mandated increased professional trustworthiness, and, hence, the need for clear ethical standards in relating to survivors. Ethical principles set the ideals for practice, and as such, give a sense of community to those who adhere to them, and to be an ethical trauma practitioner means to have a certain moral stance for self-regulation. In a broader sense, ethics and ethical codes give guidance to practice, and as such, they must be responsive, clear, grounded in fact (not fantasy), and guide practice.

Williams (2010, 2012), who developed the first code of ethics for traumatologists for the Association of Traumatic Stress Specialists in 2002, recognized the impact of trauma work on professional and personal lives, and argued that self-care is a moral obligation and professional competency of anyone who works with trauma survivors.

According to Williams, the therapist's role is to restore a survivor's capacity to trust in themselves, others, and the world, and that trauma work also can trigger countertransference, which occurs when providers have similarly unmet needs. She underscored the importance of recognizing how trauma work impacts providers, and being aware of personal and professional limitations. She further maintained that it is unethical to ignore self-care, and emphasized the role of professional competency in traumatology, which she understands as providing services within those boundaries and recognizing the limits of one's competency and capacity. Williams goes on to assert that maintaining clear boundaries between professional and personal life allows for a safe connection based on the needs of the individual being served or helped.

She approaches professional competence as a marker for good decision-making, which involves the recognition of responsibilities, personal and professional limitations, including limits of training and expertise, and providing services only within those boundaries.

5.3 Disaster Mental Health: "Hurry Up and Wait"

"Hurry up and wait" is a meme that is used in emergency response with reference to difficulties balancing two priorities, the urgency in responding to pressing needs, and the assurance of safety of the responders. For instance, De Phillis (2017) used this meme to describe the American Red Cross efforts to respond to Hurricane Harvey in Texas in 2017: "Red Cross volunteers deploying slowly, with conditions too dangerous to travel ... You know what they say about hurry up and wait?"

Jenson (1997, p. 13) who first initiated the discussion about the role of ethics in disaster management, suggested that in a disaster, the traditional tools of "objective" logic—rationality and consistency—may not be adequate. She proposed that the ethical guidelines of disaster response must be able to answer the following questions: (1) Who has the authority to make such significant ethical decisions? (2) How should ethical decisions be made—what principles and values should guide those engaged in ethical decision-making processes? (3) What is responsible action in response to human need? She emphasized that disaster management should be primarily governed by humanitarian values rather than by pursuing military or security objectives

Geale (2012) underscored the concepts of ethics and justice as important issues in disaster management. They pertain to the appropriate and fair allocation of relief funds to help with recovery; as well as to how to balance the critical need for the disaster research with the ethical obligation of respect for, and protection of, the interests of research participants. Geale (2012) goes on to identify "eight cardinal virtues of disaster response," which are prudence, courage, justice, stewardship, vigilance, resilience, self-effacing charity, and communication.

Aung, 'Inayatibt, Rahman, Nurumal, and Ahayalimudin (2017, p. 90) further noted the limitations in reliance on normative values proposing that decision-making in a disaster cannot be carried out by one person alone, or even a single community. It requires an open discussion and a commitment between the experiences and perspectives of those who are different within the affected area. Rather than asserting absolutes or providing definitive answers to the ethical dilemmas that arise in the context of disasters, the ethics of disaster response and management focus on specific aspects of disaster management that involve complex ethical issues. The people responding to disasters (victims, health care personnel, humanitarian aid workers, or military personnel) often report disillusionment and a kind of frustration with making ethical decisions during disasters, and this, according to Aung et al. (2017), confirms the pressing needs for clear ethical guidelines to help to provide stability for organizations in a rapidly changing and increasingly complex world.

To addresses these emerging concerns, the American Red Cross hires licensed MH providers to provide disaster response, meaning that disaster mental health (DMH) workers are primarily bound by their professional codes of ethics (ARC, 2017, p. 15), but also by the agency standards developed specifically for DMH. They include

- practicing in a manner that is in the best interest of the public;
- providing only those services deemed necessary;
- practicing only within the competency areas of the practitioner's education and/or experience, and maintaining the limitations established by licensure or certification;
- maintaining a confidential client–provider relationship;
- disclosing client information to others on a strict need-to-know basis;
- avoiding dual relationships with clients, whenever possible;
- refraining from personal gain due to involvement with the Red Cross, including refraining from referring Red Cross clients to their private practice/agency of employment.

5.4 Ethical Challenges in Post-Conflict Settings: What to Do with the Fish?

The term "post-conflict" does not signify the obliteration of the root causes of the outbreak of conflict in the first place. Nor does it imply a complete cessation of hostilities that often recur even after the signing of a peace agreement or the waging of elections. It frequently denotes merely an abatement of hostilities, or a "window of opportunity" for peace in a conflict that can again escalate if mismanaged (Fischer, 2004, pp. 2–3; Hamre & Sullivan, 2002, p. 90).

In humanitarian work, the mundane cliché, "if you give a man a fish, he will eat today, but teach a man to fish and he will eat forever," acquires a whole new meaning and sheds light on the complexity of factors involved in designing a helping intervention and the delicate balance between relief and sustainable solutions in post-conflict settings. Let's continue using this metaphor to further examine these matters.

First of all, while learning to fish, this person could have died of starvation. Further on, the post-conflict setting creates a whole set of new questions about

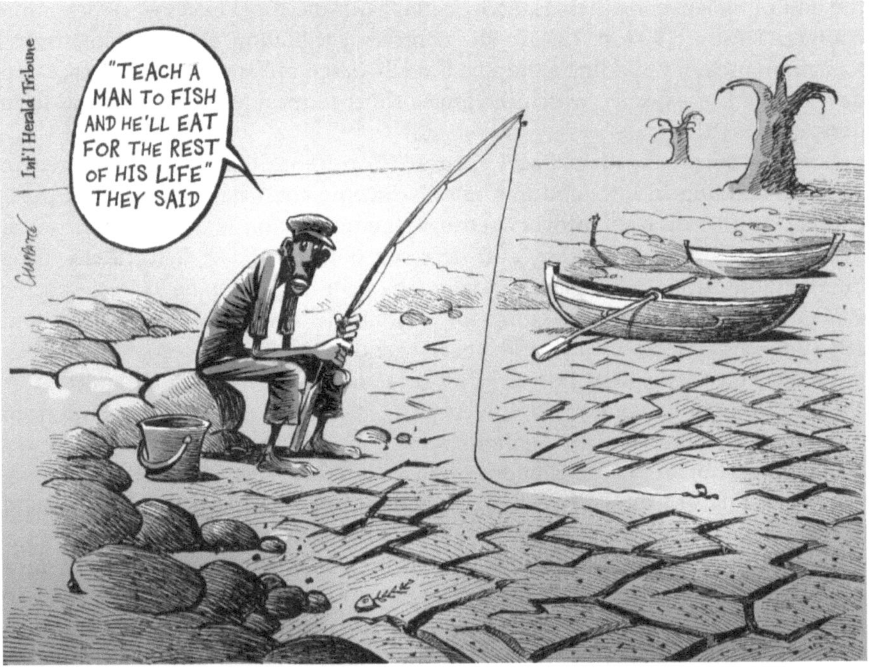

Figure 5.1 "Give Man a Fish ..." (© Chappatte in the *International New York Times*, October 23, 2009)

sustainability, equipment, and logistics. Learning how to fish won't help much without having fishing gear production in the long run. Is there a need to build the factory to produce the fishing equipment? Is there enough wood in the region to make fishing rods? But even before everything, the main question is whether fishing is sustainable or endemic to this region. Maybe there is no direct access to the large water sources or getting there is not safe; or fishing is prohibited by local culture—or maybe there are not enough fish. And, of course, there always remains the important issue: what if the neighbors who are starving use the results of this intervention as a reason to attack the "more prosperous" village? In this way, merely by trying to help, we can put the life of villagers at risk.

Figure 5.1 was initially drawn to illustrate the problem with sustainability of global resources, but I found it to be a good illustration to the described dilemma.

Transition from Relief to Recovery to Reconstruction

It has long been recognized that "quick fixes" or interventions aimed at delivering immediate relief do not necessarily create sustainable solutions. While emergency relief is often necessary to save lives, and cease-fires may be a beginning to the end of violence, neither deal adequately with the root causes of disaster and conflict (Jenson, 1997, p. 13). To the contrary, facilitation of sustainable transformation includes building a durable broadly based infrastructure for peace and development of capacity, which integrates short-term objectives with long-term perspectives (p. 16).

It is not surprising that GMH specialists are more likely to be engaged in capacity building in low- and low middle-income countries (LLMIC). In post-conflict or post-disaster recovery settings, the population is dealing with recent trauma that is compounded by daily stresses, poverty, and violence. Refocusing interventions from responsive mode to the long-term agenda brings specific challenges that include expanding the objectives to include sustainability and self-sufficiency. In an ideal world, these agendas should not compete with the immediate lifesaving goals, but in reality, the competition for resources makes this choice a point of contention. Rokhideh (2017) provided examples of solutions of how much MH interventions might impact the landscape of a complex emergency if they do factor in concerns about capacity building. For instance, developing peace-building strategies can lead to preventing violence and further suffering and trauma while fostering recovery.

While the relief modality may have clearly defined short-term goals, such as lifesaving, the objectives for MH strategies in the post-conflict setting aim to contribute to the more complex goals of long-term sustainable recovery, self-sufficiency, and violence prevention in the affected region. The following case study illustrates the systemic complexities of developing interventions in post-conflict settings.

Abramowitz (2015) demonstrates how the problem of transitioning the Liberian state from humanitarian management to a vague, ill-defined development trajectory became particularly visible in the medical sector during the early years of Liberia's post-war recovery. She called this problem "the afterlife of intervention." Rokhideh (2017) further examined the short- and long-term outcomes of psychosocial interventions in northern Uganda recovering from 22 years of civil war. According to the author, in recent years, northern Uganda saw an outpouring of humanitarian MHPSS interventions devoted to the post-conflict recovery project. Simultaneously, the region has experienced a significant rise in cases of suicides, domestic violence, substance abuse, and criminal behavior, pointing to the need to better understand the complex dynamics and experiences of everyday post-conflict life. These worrying trends drew Rokhideh (2017) to examine the extent to which the MHPSS approach has been conducive to addressing the psychosocial needs of individuals and communities in the post-conflict setting. Drawing on the public health data, reports, and interviews with providers and beneficiaries, Rokhideh (2017) demonstrated that psychosocial interventions in northern Uganda have largely (1) remained short-lived, (2) targeted specific groups at the expense of others, (3) failed to respond to the daily stressors and needs of the population, and (4) remained relatively disconnected from the wider post-conflict recovery process.

Neocolonial Agenda

Globalization and the global power differential between high-, middle-, and low-middle/low-income countries (LLMIC) has elicited concerns about using post-conflict recovery hardship for political reasons by imposing a Western agenda in *a neo-colonial* way. This term was used by Mills (2013, p. 37) in his book entitled *Decolonizing Global Mental Health: The Psychiatrization of the Majority World*, in which he sees in GMH "a form of colonialism that comes from within and from outside, swallowed in the form of a pill." These concerns reflected controversies surrounding the sensitive nature of the role of a MH agenda in multicultural contexts. Historically, the notion of "international health" has been fraught with connotations of a colonial past that stressed the "civilizatory help" of developed nations to less affluent or less medically advanced ones. The globalization of MH in post-conflict nonemergency settings intensified worries about the missionary agenda, which takes advantage of populational vulnerabilities. Watters (2010a) went on to claim that GMH carries a political agenda masked as humanitarian aid, and uses the concepts of MH for political reasons. This proposition does not appear falsifiable because it is difficult to prove one way or another, and instead we will focus on ethical challenges to the integrity of MH interventions in post-conflict settings.

The GMH critics, however, continue believing that the Western influence extends through proliferation of concepts due to power and privileges of economically developed countries, both intentionally and unintentionally. It is not a secret that the donors who provide funding do impact the programmatic decisions, which includes determining the prioritized needs. In addition, the fragmentation of funding results in fragmentation in services, which poses a problem for those who work toward building systems of care. One example of how the donors' preferences shape interventions can be when the targeted grants only fund services for female survivors of sexual violence and not for male survivors (Storr, 2011).

Whether the proliferation of the Westernization of MH concepts in LLMIC has been intentional or unintentional, these discussions mirror the concerns about the impact of globalization, which Summerfield (2002) labeled as exporting a Western model of illness and treatment that undermines the culturally appropriate traditional therapies, ignores cultural variability in comprehending and responding to mental suffering, medicalizes distress, and ignores its social and economic causes. Summerfield's (2002) advocacy posed an existential dilemma for GMH: Shall we choose to intervene if helping interventions are imperfect and come with the possibility of imposing values or way of life and foster dependence? That is leaving aside Summerfield's core belief that there is nothing the Westerners have to offer in the different culture or context.

This dilemma is depicted in the fictional universe of *Star Trek*, where the *Prime Directive* is a guiding principle of the United Federation of Planets prohibiting the protagonists from interfering with the internal development of alien civilizations. This conceptual law applies particularly to civilizations that are below a certain threshold of technological, scientific, and cultural development; preventing starship crews from using their superior technology to impose their own values or ideals on them. Peltz (2003) used this metaphor to demonstrate how a product of science fiction can be useful in understanding intercultural contacts right here on Earth. He concludes that the proper and modern-day understanding of the Prime Directive dictates that the value of cultural autonomy must be balanced with the inevitability of cultural interference and transformation. Ultimately all that the Prime Directive can teach is that when two worlds collide, people must work together to preserve the best of both (p. 635).

Earlier, Arkady and Boris Strugatsky (1965/2005), the Soviet-Russian science fiction writers, explored the connection between the power and responsibility in their novel *Hard to Be a God* in 1964. The protagonist is Anton (known as his alias Don Rumata), an undercover operative from the future planet Earth, in his mission on an alien planet that is populated by human beings whose society has not advanced beyond the Middle Ages, with all the associated violence, disease, and cruelty. He faces a moral dilemma: although he can use his advanced civilizatory knowledge to help, as an observer on the planet he is forbidden to do anything as his assistance would interfere with the natural progress of history, and any interventions could lead to unpredictable outcomes that could make the situation much worse.

These analogies are very much relevant to current concerns around the role of the well-intended GMH specialist who must exercise extreme caution not to interrupt the normal fabric of life and the natural recovery.

Cherepanov's (2015b, 2016) CBPR model was developed as an attempt to reconcile this dilemma. It proposes that MH providers are most effective when, instead of providing external intervention, they partner with the community to identify and mobilize their own recovery resources consisting of local traditions, culture, history of survivorship, and mutual supports. Building upon available resources and empowering and engaging the community helps the community to take responsibility for and invest in the recovery.

5.5 Fieldwork

GMH providers travel internationally to provide a wide range of services, interventions, and supports in complex emergency and post-conflict settings, including direct care, program management, capacity building, training local providers, and more. Clarinval and Biller-Andorno (2014) described fieldwork as a complex environment involving multiple relationships. Some of these are hierarchical, some are multidisciplinary or cross-sectional. Deciding the correct course of action can be a formidable challenge under such circumstances. Yet, decisions must be made according to professional norms and values of humanitarian action, and these decisions sometimes need to be made quickly and with consideration of their potentially very serious impacts.

Some dilemmas that GMH field workers face are unique, but most are routine and predictable, though this doesn't make their navigation any easier. In these dilemmas, as often happens in GMH, there are no right or wrong solutions as both alternatives can be equally justifiable because they represent the underlying conflict of professional paradigms. Using the desk review and drawing on my practical experience, workshops, and discussions, I identified several professional dilemmas that are commonly encountered in the fieldwork:

Dilemma 1: Obsolete Evidence-Based Practices Versus Risky Innovations

Many of the available MH assessments and "evidence-based practices" may not have been adequately validated and standardized; and some do not have relevance in the global context. Sheather et al. (2016) studied the ethical framework for humanitarian innovations and argued that the dynamic process of innovations may not fit with the conventional ethics framework, and any innovation projects introduce additional risks for populations even if human participants are not directly involved. They noted difficulties in balancing the benefits and risks of innovations with outdated practices within the professional framework and suggested using high-level principles that have been developed for humanitarian innovation, even though there is a lack of guidance for how these should be applied in practice. The authors proposed a Médecins Sans Frontières (MSF) ethics framework for humanitarian innovation and offered a self-guided decision-making algorithm for nonmedical innovators (see Table 5.2).

Dilemma 2: Immediate Needs Versus Long-Term Needs of Survivors

Rokhideh (2017) used the example of post-conflict northern Uganda to demonstrate the harm that can be caused by a failure to adjust the responsive approaches to the post-conflict setting where daily stresses exacerbate war trauma. Capacity building and facilitating systemic changes may better fit the long-term sustainable recovery goals, but may not be sufficient to meet immediate pressing needs. Prioritizing the response mode of interventions during a complex emergency is justified by their urgency. However, those who are engaged in immediate relief often can't help but wonder about the overall effectiveness of these interventions in the long run. To simplify this problem, one could question why shall we allocate resources for MH care if we are unable to save these people anyway—they are likely to get killed as a result of ongoing violence? Would it be more cost effective to invest into violence prevention or peace building instead? This is a terrible dilemma, and everyone facing it has to make very difficult decisions.

Dilemma 3: Individual Rights Versus Community Benefit

Karadag and Kerim Hakan (2012, p. 602) described this conflict between clinical and public health needs as a conflict between autonomy of the individual and the desire to protect and promote the health of the population. They believed that

Table 5.2 An MSF Ethical Framework for Humanitarian Innovations (Sheather et al., 2016)

This framework is intended to be used to guide work that does not directly involve human participants and does not lie within the purview of formal research ethics oversight.

1. Clearly *identify the problem* you are seeking to address and what benefit you expect the innovation to have. This step may seem obvious, so what is its ethical significance? When identifying the problem, there should be consideration of upstream solutions that may address the problem in a holistic and sustainable way. For instance, rather than focusing on technocratic fixes, what are the sociopolitical determinants of the problem and the wider possibilities for solutions? Who has stakes in finding a solution and who may have interests in perpetuating the problem? Is the problem a moving target? Collaboration and cross-fertilization with other disciplines should be considered in order to help to see the problem from various perspectives. In short, do not underestimate the importance of fully identifying the problem.
2. *Ensure that the innovation shows respect for human dignity*. While this is a broad concept, it has practical implications. The focus of concern is respect for human beings, reminding us that the simplest or most direct solutions may not be ethically appropriate. Innovators must show due respect for the multiple and overlapping interests of those affected by the innovation. This extends beyond a concern for physical well-being to include psychological and cultural integrity. It also incorporates a concern for individual privacy and a respect for the confidentiality of individual, family, and community-based data.
3. *Clarify how you will involve the end user* from the beginning of the process. Innovation should be driven by the requirements of the user. The innovation cycle should be participatory, using methods to involve relevant individuals and communities. Innovators must be sensitive to power dynamics between and within cultures as well as power imbalances between aid workers and beneficiaries.
4. *Identify and weigh harms and benefits*. When considering innovations, a critical first step is the identification, as far as is reasonably possible, of potential harms along with the anticipated benefits. The next step involves weighing these harms and benefits.
   a. Where reasonably foreseeable harms outweigh the likely benefits, implementation will not be ethical. Potential harms include, but are not limited to, physical and psychological harm to individuals. There is also a need to consider any potential harm to communities.
   b. Where innovation involves a favorable balance of benefits and harms, all reasonable steps must be taken to minimize (mitigate) the harms as far as possible. Unnecessary harms must be eliminated. Where harms are unavoidable, those affected should be informed of the nature and severity of the risks involved.
   c. Conflicted partnerships or conflicts of interest may result in reputational harm to the organization. If these are identified, then oversight by an existing ethics review board is recommended.
5. *Describe the distribution of harms and benefits, and ensure that the risk of harm is not borne by those who do not stand to benefit*. Innovators need to give careful consideration to the distribution of benefits and harms associated with their projects. Do the risks or benefits fall unequally across groups? If so, is it appropriate to proceed, and how can these inequalities of distribution be addressed or mitigated? Equally, it is important that the innovation take into account vulnerable groups; it may be ethically warranted to give particular attention to those who have particular needs. Just as we tend to give more health care to the unwell, so particular attention may need to be given to those

Table 5.2 (Cont.)

who are vulnerable or who may not be able to protect their own interests. This is expressed in the humanitarian principle of impartiality. In addition, consider whether anyone is "wronged" by the innovation. A "wrong" is an infringement that is distinct from harm. For example, selecting one group for an innovation project over another may wrong the other group (as opposed to harming them).
6. *Plan (and carry out) an evaluation that delivers the information needed for subsequent decisions to implement or scale up the innovation; then ensure that the beneficiaries have access to the innovation.* Innovation requires an acceptance of the risk of failure—not all innovation projects will achieve their desired outcome. But in all cases, we can learn and apply these lessons in the future. Given the time, energy, and resources that these projects require, rigorous evaluation and sharing of lessons is itself a moral obligation. Therefore, consideration should be given to the dissemination of findings, since it may be important to avoid further exposure to potential harm by sharing findings, whether these are positive or negative. Likewise, there should be a willingness and strategy for wider implementation of the innovation if found to be successful, and a commitment to ensure that beneficiaries—at least in the communities where it was tested and ideally in similar communities affected by humanitarian crises—subsequently have access to the innovation.

emergency settings require stronger effort to achieve a balance between individual and collective rights. An example of such a dilemma can be a decision whether to quarantine an individual who shows symptoms of a contagious disease. While this may seem to benefit this person who would receive treatment, and this measure could prevent further spread of the disease, the community may respond by hiding their infected family members preventing them from being taken to the medical compound where "everyone dies"—which, contrary to the initial intent, may lead to an increased spread of the infection. Finding practical solutions for this dilemma was extremely important during the Ebola outbreak in West Africa, where setting up the quarantine in Monrovia resulted in increased distrust and hostility toward the medical providers, community tensions, and hiding infected patients (E. Cherepanov, personal communication, August 30, 2014).

Another facet of the conflict between individual and public interests is the "loose lips sink ships" dilemma. In this dilemma, a provider who decides to engage in *temoignage* (testimony) for a minority group must take into consideration that the exposure and advocacy may expose them to a greater danger, or to being used by a government to oust the humanitarian aid organizations from the region.

Dilemma 4: Extensive Needs of Affected Populations Versus Limited Resources

This dilemma I call "how to measure suffering," or how to decide who most needs help. Needs assessments help to set the priorities, but in the field when there is so much human suffering, this dilemma can present a daily professional and personal struggle. Funding, human resources, logistics, and personal capacity place limitations on what providers can do and who they help, and having to turn away those who need help goes against our human nature and puts a heavy emotional burden on the providers.

Dilemma 5: Planned Interventions Versus Impromptu Interventions

This dilemma reflects a conflict between programmatic demands and the mandate and unplanned challenges. In the field, where planning is a cornerstone for consistent and coordinated efforts, self-determination, flexibility, and "thinking outside of the box" are often needed to respond to the needs of the volatile and rapidly changing situation. Finding the right balance between planning and improvisation so that it does not undermine the project's goals can be a challenging task. This dilemma is often a source of major frustration when remotely positioned managers insist on their recommendations being followed exactly, and it is not easy to know whether they lack appreciation for the dynamics on the ground or if they are considering the bigger picture (E. Cherepanov, personal communication, November 20, 2015).

Dilemma 6: Institutional Values Versus Professional or Personal Values

It is not uncommon when the professional's understanding of their role conflicts with the institutional values or expectations. Organizational and professional beliefs can diverge drastically regarding attitudes toward birth control when supporting rape victims, stances on *temoignage*, or over contentions as slight as what methods and interventions to use. These dilemmas indicate the importance of clarifying the institutional values prior to the deployment and checking them against personal and professional values; this can boil down to the question of whether MH providers can work with the NGO whose ground values or religious affiliation they do not share. And if yes, how much they can concede their own principles or convictions in exchange for the opportunity to help others?

Dilemma 7: Is It Okay to Wave Ethical Standards to Gain Access to the Population in Need?

An example of this dilemma can be when local officials demand bribes in exchange for allowing the health care providers to gain access to the affected region. The other facet of this dilemma pertains to reported cases where providers have paid people to participate in different activities, such as attending psychoeducation sessions (Bobkoff, 2016). In the National Public Radio podcast, Warner (2017) examined the controversial attempts to address rape in the Congo, which resulted in an increase in false claims to get access to benefits. Can not-so-perfect screenings be warranted if they make it easier for genuine rape survivors to gain access to services? Should we pay the beneficiaries to receive vaccinations or to participate in psychoeducation, treatment, or research? These dilemmas are indicative of the contextual complexity of many problems in a humanitarian context, underlying the importance that the decisions are made collaboratively and are supported by their deploying agency that hopefully had carefully researched all the options and consequences.

5.6 Case Study Exercise: Navigating Ethical Dilemmas in Fieldwork

The case studies offered below provide an opportunity to discuss and practice strategies for navigating dilemmas arising in fieldwork. Some examples are hypothetical cases, while others are loosely based on real scenarios.

Instructions

- Read the case scenario.
- Identify the professional dilemma(s).
- Determine whether there is a conflict of values.
- Describe the benefits and disadvantages of prioritizing one conflicting value over another.
- Discuss how would you resolve the dilemma.

Case Study 1

Soon after the devastating 2010 earthquake in Haiti, MH professionals traveled there to provide psychosocial support. The sheer number of severely traumatized citizens, complicated by the language barrier and scarcity of interpreters, greatly impeded the use of conventional trauma therapy. Instead, MH professionals started using Thought Field Therapy, the nonverbal energy approach that at the time was not endorsed by the APA.[1] The providers experimented with using this method on large groups and reported that the participants found the experience extremely helpful. Even now, many years later, elements of TFT still continue to be incorporated into recovery programs, such as rhythmic dance movements as part of art therapy modules (E. Cherepanov, personal communication, November 20, 2016).

What would you do? Would you use this approach or decide against it? What can be the benefits or concerns of either decision?

Case Study 2

In a remote African village, a MH provider notices a woman who is tied to a tree. When the husband says that this woman is mentally ill, the provider asserts her human rights and demands that she be freed. The husband explains that in the village, there is no access to psychiatrists or medications. They know that tying is bad, but if they set her free, she would wander into the bushes and get lost, or end up beaten or raped. The family is unable to watch her all the time because they have to work.

"What do you suggest I do?" he asks.

Case Study 3

During the Ebola outbreak in West Africa in 2015, attempts to quarantine those who were infected resulted in the reluctance of family members to inform public health authorities, often hiding those who may have contracted the disease. In the course of your work, a patient trusts you, the MH provider, enough to disclose that a family member has been displaying symptoms of an infectious disease, and begs you to keep it a secret.

What would you do? What can be the consequences of the decisions?

Case Study 4

In a refugee camp, a MH provider who works in a medical compound where there are sick patients sees a man being chased by a mob of camp residents, who claim that they recognized him as a war criminal. The man approaches the compound and begs for asylum.

What would you do? What can be the consequences of the decisions?

Case Study 5

A participant requests payment for attending the psychoeducation groups.

Would your decision be different if this is vaccination?

What would you do? What can be the consequences of either decision?

Note

1 The APA removed the ban on continuing education for energy psychology only in 2012, adding it to the National Registry of Evidence-Based Programs and Practices (National Psychologist Staff. July 27, 2016).

CHAPTER 6

Aspirational Guidance: Principles of Humanitarian Assistance

6.1 Fundamental Principles of Humanitarian Assistance

Fidelity to humanitarian principles is the backbone of GMH. These principles remind us of the reasons why this profession exists, and set its moral compass. As Rysaback-Smith (2015, p. 7) wrote, the humanitarian principles must always remain at the forefront of provision of aid especially now when humanitarians' work becomes increasingly complex and the international conflicts and disasters are more frequent and increasingly geopolitical.

The values that govern humanitarian work have been developed over time and continue to incorporate the experiences of humanitarian action and emerging challenges. Throughout their evolution, however, the fundamental principles of humanitarian assistance have remained the aspiration and defining characteristics of multi-disciplinary humanitarianism.

As indicated in Chapter 2, the history of the universal humanitarian values dates back to 1965 when the International Federation of the Red Cross (IFRC, 1965) formulated their Fundamental Principles of the Movement, which were humanity, impartiality, independence, and neutrality. Later, the list of principles has expanded and included the humanitarian imperative, accountability, and transparency. Following certain highly publicized incidents, principles against exploiting vulnerabilities were added. This demonstrates that the humanitarian values are a continual work in progress that reflects the positive and problematic experience of the humanitarian community, where the measure of success is alleviation of suffering and saving human lives. While the exact wording of the principles varies slightly across NGOs, they are all built upon respect for human rights, transparency, and accountability.

Harris (2013) made the important distinction between preventative or regulatory ethics, which consist of guidelines for preventing harm to the public, and aspirational ethics, which consist of guidelines and motivating considerations for the use of professional expertise, and called for an increase in prominence for aspirational ethics. Candilis and Martinez (2006) echo this position stating that aspirational ideals set a higher standard for professionals than any minimalist legal requirement because they provide a morally protective presence. In the context of the humanitarian work, the aspirational guidance is provided by the universal humanitarian principles that establish the professional values of integrity, honesty, truth, and fairness and keeps us true to the ideals for the profession we want it to be.

Aspirational values provide motivational considerations for ensuring universal human rights in complex environments fraught with controversy, political battles, and multidisciplinary values. They also set the directionality or moral compass for such interventions. Hilhorst (2005), however, pointed out their limitations in the area of proactive regulation or in seeking guidance, and for purposes of accountability (p. 364). She described the aspirational guidance as "we shall endeavor to" instead of "we shall," which means that humanitarian values organize decision-making but do not ensure the result.

It is important to note that some organizations that label their work as humanitarian assistance, such as military forces and for-profit companies, are not considered humanitarian agencies, and they are not obliged to base their interventions on these principles. Working with such organizations places more responsibility on the MH specialist in clarifying their professional role and organizational values prior to deployment.

To summarize the findings in the literature, the role of humanitarian principles in GMH as a humanitarian profession is to:

- provide aspirational guidance and professional ideals;
- set the system of higher level values to navigate conflicts of professional values;
- establish a broad meta-level frame of reference that is shared by multidisciplinary and cross-sectional humanitarian actors;
- flag practices that violate human rights and undermine the humanitarian spirit.

6.2 Humanitarian Principles as Aspirational Guidance: A Moral Compass

In their work, GMH providers will likely face dilemmas where any decision comes with a serious cost. In the context of uncertainty and conflicting values, the humanitarian principles provide a meta-level reference and offer strategic guidance for such decision-making.

While Hillhorst (2005, p. 364) viewed the humanitarian principles that are reflected in the NGO's Code of Conduct as a comprehensive and appropriate instrument for discussing operational matters, I argue that while humanitarian principles set ideals that the profession strives to achieve, they do not directly translate into the operations. Furthermore, using the aspirations as operational guidance has created such undertakings as "humanitarian military operations" or historical enterprises such as totalitarian regimes where the humanitarian ideals were used to justify social experiments. For example, the 1917 October Revolution in Russia (the 100-year anniversary of which we celebrate this year) had its inspiration in the most "idealistic" ideals *of justice*, *equity*, and *liberty* (Kreitman, 1996), resultant in a humanitarian catastrophe.

Next, the humanitarian values will be described using the principles of humanitarian assistance adopted by the IFRC (1965/1994). The following discussion points and the hypothetical examples outline gray areas and ambiguities that arise when we approach principles as operational guidance.

Humanitarian Principles

1. The Humanitarian Imperative

The *humanitarian imperative* is a core principle of humanity that means that all humankind shall be treated humanely and equally in all circumstances by saving lives and alleviating suffering, while ensuring respect for the individual.

Discussion

The humanitarian imperative has been recognized by the Sphere Project (2004) as a governing principle of the humanitarian chapter, where nothing should override this principle. It is important, however, to recognize that the humanitarian imperative can be affected by external constraints: sometimes it can be an intervention of convenience. Using this principle in determining the prioritized needs inadvertently leads to the brutal dilemma: How can we prioritize those who are in greater need of MH support? Who do we help first? Is it at all possible to measure or compare suffering? The strong potential for real or perceived injustice in setting humanitarian priorities and arising moral dilemmas suggests a need for further guidance in justification of interventions when the choices are limited or predetermined by external forces (donors' expectations, institutional priorities, political or security contexts). An important part of this decision-making is to decide whether doing something that may be unjust is better than doing nothing.

2. The Humanitarian Accountability Principle

The *humanitarian accountability principle* means that "we [i.e. humanitarians] hold ourselves accountable to both those we seek to assist and those from whom we accept resources" (IFRC, 1965/1994), which can be understood as an imperative to use power responsibly and balance the needs of stakeholders with a commitment to providing assistance (Lloyd et al., 2005, p. 5). The IASC (2007) guidelines added that accountability also involves avoiding unnecessary and costly redundancies and focusing on response, sustainable development, and local capacity building.

Discussion

For MH specialists, accountability underscores the paramount importance of professional competencies, commitment to the professional code of ethics, and adherence to the principles of humanitarian work. It also means carrying the highest degree of personal and professional integrity and responsibility for the consequences of helping interventions, both intended and unintended. However, the execution of this principle opens up questions: Are there any limits to professional responsibility toward the people we serve and the organizations we work with? What are they? Who are we primarily accountable to if the needs of clientele and the organization or funder conflict? And finally, how can we be responsible for the consequences of helping interventions when it is nearly impossible to predict the outcome in the volatile context of a humanitarian emergency?

Another side of accountability is about deciding who are we accountable to: donors, affected population, or the organizations, which includes the professional bodies. This approach to understanding the accountability leads to even tougher questions. What if these accountabilities collide and what is good for donors may not be good for the affected population? How can we decide for the people what they need? And how do we reconcile our understanding of their needs with the agency's agenda or availability of the resources? Accountability is discussed further in section 6.3 below.

3. Impartiality

The principle of *impartiality* requires that provision of humanitarian assistance must be impartial and not based on nationality, race, religion, or political point of view. It must be based on need alone.

Discussion

Although it is hardly realistic to expect absolute impartiality from a MH professional as a human being who is working with survivors of armed conflict, a self-awareness of personal bias is a good beginning to managing cognitive distortions and establishing impartial care. At the same time, providing MH supports to both (or all) sides of a conflict can amplify the tensions and resentment within the community, complicate access to survivors, and put providers at further risk. For example, treating perpetrators and the survivors in the same hospital or by the same providers can leave all of them feeling unsafe. Impartiality in programmatic implementation may also be significantly challenged by the political context when decisions about the nature of the program and target population are based on the available funding, and the funders do not feel the obligation to be impartial. Furthermore, fundraising opportunities depend on media exposure that is often biased towards one side of the conflict. What stance should we as the professionals take if the funders or the organizational values are not impartial? And finally, is a partial intervention better than no intervention at all?

4. Independence

The principle of *independence* stipulates that humanitarian agencies must formulate and implement their own policies independent of government policies or actions.

Discussion

The independence principle emphasizes that the NGO alone must decide who and when to help, independent of governments. At the same time, the effectiveness of aid, sustainability of recovery, and safety of the people we serve to a large degree depends on building upon available infrastructure, as well as developing collaborations with governments and public health establishments when possible. Balancing this independence with capacity building is always a delicate act. The other facet of the independence principle pertains to the role of a GMH professional. How far can we go in debating the independence? Can the individual or group of professionals formulate their own policies and values? What if these values conflict with those established by the NGO or professional organization they belong to?

5. Neutrality

The *neutrality* principle prohibits humanitarians taking sides in a conflict or engaging at any time in controversies of a political, racial, religious, or ideological nature.

Discussion

This is probably the most contentious principle. It was initially developed to assert the precedence of international humanitarian law in events of armed conflict. This principle has been met with apprehension because some believe that the principle of neutrality conflicts with promoting social justice and advocating for social or political change, which are important parts of GMH work—as Chomsky (1999) once said: "neutrality in the face of murder is immoral." The contradiction of this principle with the *temoignage* that NGOs have felt bound by eventually led to the creation of Médecins Sans Frontières (MSF, 1971), which believed the world needed to know about the events they were witnessing, and that has proposed that solidarity replace the neutrality principle. For the MSF mission *temoignage* is a central principle of the organization and also that it is the responsibility of MSF to speak out and bring attention to humanitarian issues that are not being addressed or are being inadequately addressed (MSF, 2011). However, this position has been challenged by Redfield (2008) who believes that any humanitarian act must also be a political act, an act in opposition to the current system that has led to human suffering, and who doesn't see a humanitarian action without politics.

6. Not Exploiting Vulnerabilities

a) *Proselytizing.* This principle states that the provision of aid must not exploit the vulnerability of victims nor be used to further political or religious creeds.

Discussion

Even this seemingly obvious principle of not exploiting vulnerability can easily become a gray area in fieldwork. The awareness of the dynamics of power and control in MH fieldwork helps to minimize the risks of purposefully or inadvertently exploiting those we are trying to help. At the same time: Is it realistic to expect that a MH provider can fully control how they and their work are perceived? What if the program is funded by a religious mission? And how do we prevent the provider's self-disclosure of personal beliefs, religious affiliation, or political views from being impressed upon the beneficiaries? Where do we draw the line? Can MH providers be responsible for how their work or faith are perceived, used, or misused by a third party when a project is funded by a faith-based or politically engaged NGO?

b) *Sexual exploitation*. This principle proclaims that sexual exploitation and abuse by humanitarian workers constitute acts of gross misconduct.

Discussion

Humanitarian agencies are responsible for developing codes of conduct that prevent abuse of the beneficiaries. This implies that humanitarian workers are not to take advantage of the vulnerabilities of those affected by war, violence, or famine. This principle is the imperative and not the aspiration, and there are no circumstances where it can be flexed or misunderstood. In an emergency where victims have lost everything, they are particularly vulnerable to sexual abuse (Gillan & Moszynski, 2002; Wall, 2016), and this addendum was developed in response to a number of reports that identified the sexual exploitation by UN and non-UN personnel of refugees in Africa, Haiti, and other regions. The fact that not all of these allegations were later substantiated (Gillan & Moszynski, 2002) only emphasizes that not only must humanitarians not engage in unethical actions but they also must avoid leaving the impression of possible impropriety.

6.3 Humanitarian Accountability or "Nothing About Us Without Us"

Accountability

Accountability is a principle that fosters responsibility of humanitarian organizations to provide services of high quality and integrity, and this principle has become a central theme in the modern humanitarianism. The International Humanitarian Accountability Partnership (HAP) was established in 2003 to promote accountability when working with people affected by humanitarian crises. HAP (2010, p. 9) developed the "Standards in Humanitarian Accountability and Quality Management," which was the first international standard designed to assess, improve, and recognize the accountability and quality of humanitarian programs. It asserted that accountability is mandatory for organizations that assist or act on behalf of people affected by disasters, conflict, poverty, or other crises because such organizations exercise significant power to save lives and reduce suffering. In contrast, crisis-affected people have no formal control, and often little influence, over these organizations. As a result, it is difficult for those people to hold organizations responsible for actions taken on their behalf. Being accountable to people they help, requires organizations to develop quality programs that meet those people's needs, and reduces the possibility of mistakes, abuse, and corruption. In this context, the HAP Standards help organizations to assess, improve, and recognize the quality and accountability of their work and benefit both the organizations and the people affected by crises.

In 2014, the IFRC confirmed adoption of the Accountability Framework methodology, which places *respect* at the center of the accountability paradigm. Under this model, respect is vital for the acceptance of the humanitarians' presence by host governments, for their ability to access beneficiaries, and for maintaining support from their donors. IFRC defined accountability as an ongoing process that creates relationships of respect between an organization and those affected by its work. In being accountable, one fulfills a commitment to enable and facilitate stakeholders to assess one's actions against defined commitments and expectations, and to respond to the assessment appropriately. In the IFRC model, four key conditions must be observed to ensure accountability:

- *Setting expectations.* We clarify what stakeholders can expect from us and the methods by which we can be assessed.
- *Information disclosure.* We actively allow stakeholders to access information necessary to make an assessment.
- *Stakeholder evaluation.* We support stakeholders in assessing the organization.
- *Learning and improvement.* We consider assessments and make appropriate changes and responses.

The IFRC uses the wheel of accountability model to ensure a unified approach by the IFRC and national societies and to achieve best practices in the field of accountability, while taking into consideration different members' contexts.

"Nothing About Us Without Us"

While there is the evident interest of the humanitarian community toward the concept of accountability, its exact meaning has not been so clear. Tan and von Schreeb (2015) reviewed a total of 85 articles and found four main themes used to define accountability: empowering aid recipients; being in an optimal position to do the greatest good; meeting expectations; and being liable. They concluded that the concept was defined poorly in many organizations and that there was a wide variation in the interpretation and understanding of accountability in the humanitarian context. This finding places a greater responsibility on providers, NGOs, and the profession to identify what accountability means for them and how it can be measured.

De Torrente and Stobbaerts (2008) shared the observation that, while there is no question that humanitarian organizations must be accountable, "accountability" has been becoming a global buzzword without a clearly defined concept, and they formulated the core questions around accountability, which were: accountable to whom, about what, and for what purpose? They identified at least three different strands in their conceptualization of accountability:

1. Focus on setting general or technical standards.
2. Results- and outcomes-oriented management, and the certification of (humanitarian) organizations that comply with set norms and processes.
3. A rights-based approach, positing that humanitarian organizations have obligations, particularly toward those they aim to help (accountability to beneficiaries).

De Torrente and Stobbaerts (2008) further argued that not listening to those caught up in conflict can result in a stereotypical response that fits our preconceived notions of the "ideal" or powerless victim and the organizational priorities rather than actual, pressing needs, where those who speak for the community frequently have little interest in those who most need help. For instance, the detection and treatment of sexual violence, a critical yet largely invisible need, can be effective only if women actively seek out help.

Crittenden (2016) referred to this lesson as "nothing about us without us"—a principle initially formulated by disability rights advocates. In humanitarian action, this principle means that affected communities are best suited to evaluate the feasibility of solutions offered on their behalf and should be fully engaged as co-creators. Crittenden provides examples of effective community engagement in planning interventions, which include the American Red Cross' collaborative project for deploying wireless sensor networks for fire detection in Nairobi's informal settlements.

Martin Fellenz (2017), a specialist in organizational behavior, stated that "Too little accountability creates monsters; too much blame creates fools." He argued that externally imposed top-down accountability does not work as intended. He proposed that the quicker and more deliberately accountability moves from evaluation to understanding to learning, the more value it creates. In his opinion, effective accountability systems and practices have three time orientations: the past (to understand and learn), the future (to design effective systems and approaches), and the present (to guide effective and appropriate behavior).

If we are to apply this strategy to the GMH domain, it would mean that (1) building the systems of accountability should be based on examining past achievements and shortfalls, identification of the areas that require further development, and standards to guide the decision-making; and (2) accountability is not equal to micromanagement and needs to be rooted in values to encompass the complexity of humanitarian work.

6.4 Exercise: Using an Aspirational Framework for Decision-Making

Goal

The goal of this exercise is to practice using humanitarian values as aspirations for decision-making. As demonstrated in this chapter, aspirations do not directly translate into operational guidance but rather set the ideals. Because humanitarian values are such an important part of professional identity and determine the image of the profession, the interventions must not only be just, transparent, and fair, but also appear as such to the stakeholders. The proposed four-step road map can be used to navigate programmatic decisions and to calibrate them to assure their consistency with the spirit of humanitarianism. Each step comes with decision-guiding questions.

Instructions

Read the hypothetical case scenarios and follow the four-step road map to decide on actions so that they do not contradict the humanitarian principles. Justify how the intervention is consistent with humanitarian principles. Adjust the intervention, if needed.

1. *Humanitarian principles.* Is the proposed intervention consistent with the spirit of humanitarian principles, and does it carry the potential for a conflict of values?
2. *Accountability.* Identify to whom the providers are primarily accountable. Is there a conflict of accountabilities?
3. *Safety or lesser harm.* Is safety at risk? What solution brings less harm: to implement the intervention or decide against it?
4. *Justification and injustice reduction.* Are the interventions transparent, fair, and just, and do they appear as such? How can the decision about the choice of interventions be justified for funders, stakeholders, and the community?

Example

A provider received a grant to set up an art therapy program for a group of children in the refugee camp. The project can accommodate 20 children. In the meantime, there are many other children who could benefit from this intervention. In addition, specialists brought with them snacks and colorful supplies that make participation in the group very attractive. Rumors swirl in the community that there is bribery involved in the selection of participants, and parents have started bringing food and valuables.

Discussion

1. *Humanitarian principles as aspiration.* Superficially, the suggested intervention appears to conflict with the Humanitarian Imperative because the target

group is chosen based on funding and resources, not on sheer need. Although the providers may not have flexibility in designing the program, the criteria for selecting children needs to be clear and thought through ahead of time. The scores on the questionnaire, for example, can serve as such criteria.

2. *Accountability.* The community has not been engaged in designing the project, nor was it consulted about how this project can best meet the community needs. Lack of community support for the project adversely affects the psychological recovery of the participants and their community re-integration.
3. *Safety or lesser harm.* Discussion about cost-benefits can help answer the questions about what brings less harm—to provide an intervention that appears unjust or to decide against it. It seems like, even if this limited intervention cannot help all the children, it will help some. However, the problematic project implementation may increase risks for the participants and the providers.
4. *Justification and injustice reduction.* The criteria for selection of children must be fair, just, and transparent to the community to avoid accusations of corruption and to prevent jealousy toward participating children. Community leaders should be involved in this communication. To reduce the perceived injustice, some fun activities for the community and small gifts can be offered to other children who weren't selected to participate in the project.

Case Scenarios for Practice

Scenario 1

MH providers are working in a region that is torn by sectorial violence. In their work, they learn about the atrocities committed by one side of the conflict and feel that *temoignage* is important to increase awareness about the conflict. Survivors say that they are afraid of the backlash if the ruling government learns about their complaints. It is also possible that in this case you may not be allowed to continue your work.

Scenario 2

A MH provider who is frustrated with the lack of progress in treating rape survivors empowers them to address the rape culture in the community, to stand up for themselves, and to confront the perpetrators.

Scenario 3

The salary of a staff interpreter who is a local personnel is far lower than the salary of expats. He requests equal pay.

Scenario 4

A MH worker wants to sponsor the education of a teenager in the community.

Scenario 5
You are the only MH provider in the region and have no expertise or mandate to work with survivors of gender-based violence. You are asked to help rape victims who are in great need of psychosocial supports.

Scenario 6
Community members inform a GMH professional that a coworker is romantically involved with a local woman who is not a client, promising her that he will bring her to his country.

Scenario 7
A village soccer team is preparing for a match against a neighboring community, which is a big deal and makes everybody excited. A MH provider wants to donate equipment to their team.

Scenario 8
A fundraiser or journalist asks you to take photos of suffering victims because this will help to raise money for their help.
What about taking photos of providers in the work environment?
What about taking selfies with the survivors?

Scenario 9
When passing by the local market, a provider encounters a family selling their family jewelry for a little money or food. The provider is interested to buy them.

Scenario 10
Local administrations allow psychosocial and health services in the community in exchange for "donations."
What if this allows access to survivors under the condition that no information is disclosed outside of the community?
What if the government would allow MH providers to access the survivors of sectarian violence only if they also treat the governmental armed forces?

Scenario 11
A community leader wants to be paid for endorsing a community educational event on de-stigmatization of MH issues.
What about paying the participants for attendance?
What about offering them food for their attendance?

CHAPTER 7

Operational Guidance: IASC Guidelines

7.1 IASC Core Principles: Consistency and Coordination

As was established in Chapter 6, the fundamental principles of humanitarian assistance provide aspirational guidance, and the IASC guidelines (IASC, 2007) lay out the operational framework for mental health and psychosocial supports (MHPSS) in increasingly complex humanitarian environments. Rysaback-Smith (2015) describes this environment as being fraught with controversy, political battles, and multiple international organizations, and Cherepanov (2017a) sees the role of ethics as ensuring that supports and interventions are implemented in a way that is consistent with both humanitarian and professional values.

Humanitarian values provide aspirational directionality, similar to how a marine compass points the direction of where to go in the sea, but the operational guidelines instruct the operators on how to sail to get there. In designing and implementing the programs, operational guidance establishes architecture and the means for intervention and ensure adherence to professional standards, integrity, and efficiency of interventions. To paraphrase Candilis and Martinez (2006), the aspirational values honor ideals and moral presence where the operational guidelines acknowledge duty.

The crucial importance of consistency and coordination in humanitarian action has long been acknowledged. It first became apparent to the humanitarian community in the wake of the Ethiopian famine of the 1980s, after massive media exposure revealed fragmented, uncoordinated humanitarian relief efforts (Sphere Project, 2004). Inadequate, scattered, and sometimes competing services when various agencies rush (they call it "flocking") to a disaster site without much regard to safety protocols or already established services can be confusing and damaging to the survivors, especially when providers use different models or offer contradicting recommendations. It also does a disservice to the image of the profession as something that survivors can trust. Needless to say, the development of collaborations among agencies providing MH services has proven to be a daunting task (Cherepanov, 2016).

In this context, the Interagency Standing Committee (IASC, 2007) undertook the challenging task of establishing operational standards for mental health and psychosocial supports (MHPSS) to facilitate the integration of different modules into coordinated humanitarian relief. The IASC has been working on developing strategic priorities for psychosocial operations in emergency settings since the 1970s, and in 2007 they issued their recommendations for the targeted psychosocial module, which has become a gold standard of humanitarian action.

As stated, the IASC's *Guidelines for Mental Health and Psychosocial Support in Emergency Settings* (2007) were developed to provide intersectoral operational consistency. The guidelines are grouped into six core principles for implementing psychosocial interventions, which translate into 25 actions clustered in three domains: emergency preparedness, minimum responses, and comprehensive responses. The scope of service that was defined by operational principles aimed to enable multidisciplinary humanitarian actors to plan and coordinate interventions and implement them in a coordinated manner. At the same time, the IASC has recognized the limitations of the operational guidelines and cautioned against using them "as a cookbook" (p. 9), emphasizing that it contains key actions but their practical implementation requires further considerations.

7.2 The Role of Ethics in Operations

The IASC guidelines (2007) aimed to reconcile multidisciplinary and intersectoral agendas, setting professional standards for planning, and implementing MH and psychosocial interventions, or "what to do." Whereas the ethical guidance refers to "how to do it right" and "what not to do."

In implementing the operational guidelines, the role of ethics is to:

- establish strategies for planning and implementation of the interventions;
- set priorities in operational decision-making if multidisciplinary or multi-layered professional values conflict;
- set standards for professional decision-making based on prioritized professional and humanitarian values;
- set a point of reference in situations with moral ambiguities;
- flag unethical practices, or "what not to do";
- prioritize safety imperatives, self-awareness, and self-care.

This chapter will examine the six core principles and how they are described in the IASC guidelines (2007, pp. 9–11): human rights and equity, participation, do no harm, building on available resources and capacities, integrated support systems, and multilayered supports. The operational principles listed below are followed with a discussion about the ethical challenges in their implementation when the guidelines can conflict with the demands of fieldwork. Mapping these areas helps to develop operational strategies that are professional, situation-congruent, and flexible.

Human Rights and Equity

> Humanitarian actors should promote the human rights of all affected persons and protect individuals and groups who are at heightened risk of human rights violations. Humanitarian actors should also promote equity and non-discrimination.
>
> (IASC, 2007, p. 9)

This principle references the universal human rights and impartiality, which state that a psychosocial provider shall make no discrimination as to nationality, race, religious beliefs, class, or political opinions. It endeavors to alleviate suffering of individuals, being guided solely by their needs, and to give priority to the most urgent cases of distress (IFRC, 1965). Using this principle for operational guidance provokes a series of difficult questions:

- How do we decide who has greater needs if we have to choose?
- Is our primary mission as professionals to promote human rights *or* to alleviate suffering? What if these agendas conflict and relief from suffering comes at the price of abandoning human rights? Which value do we prioritize, for example, in a situation when access to a suffering population is conditioned upon establishing collaboration with the regime known for violating human rights? Or another scenario: Where do we draw the line when pursuing human rights places people at risk, as can happen when advocacy exposes vulnerable groups?
- How realistic it is to expect true impartiality in conducting interventions that are funded by potentially partial donors?
- Is it better to plan interventions in a potentially unjust way or not do anything at all? And if there are objective limitations in interventions, how can aid professionals justify the choice for the affected population, international community, and to themselves?

Balancing this principle and the demands of fieldwork can be particularly challenging when operational decisions are largely based on the availability of resources, funding, or the mission of the NGO. Quite commonly, the decision about who needs help first is determined by the political and media prominence of the issue. One example of this selectiveness is the NGOs' approach to pervasive sexual violence against men. Patrick's (2011) article in the *Atlantic* challenged international nongovernmental organizations (INGOs) and the United Nations (UN) for "barely acknowledging" this problem, instead diverting those resources designated for gender-based violence exclusively to females. The article documented that

22 percent of men in East Congo reported being victims of sexual violence, compared to 30 percent of women, and that those men had received little or no attention from the INGO community.

These ambiguities with operationalizing this principle hint at its aspirational nature, which means that it must be used for operational guidance with great caution. I suggest the criterion that allows differentiation between aspirational and operational values: If the practical use of the guideline creates more ambiguities than it brings solutions, it points to its aspirational quality. The aspirational role of *human rights and equity* questions the conceptual homogeneity and overall benefits of listing this principle within the same group as other IASC operational guidelines.

Participation

> Humanitarian action should maximize the participation of local affected populations in the humanitarian response. In most emergency situations, significant numbers of people exhibit sufficient resilience to participate in relief and reconstruction efforts.
>
> (IASC, 2007, p. 10)

This principle serves to promote independence and self-reliance. It emphasizes the active role that survivors play in their psychological and social recovery. Far from suggesting that the professional opinion does not matter, this principle can be best served when the affected population is engaged in decision-making. Recently, this principle acquired additional meaning within the context of the push for the accountability. Crittenden (2016) described it as "nothing about us without us"—a principle initially introduced by the disability rights movement. In humanitarian action, this principle means that involving the affected communities in planning interventions allows them to be fully engaged as co-creators of their recovery. At the same time, some strategies stemming from this approach have recently attracted sharp criticism after the facts emerged about controversial practices such as paying participants for engaging in conversation about education or counseling needs and for attending the sessions (Bobkoff, 2016).

Do No Harm

> Work on mental health and psychosocial support has the potential to cause harm because it deals with highly sensitive issues.
>
> (IASC, 2007, p. 10)

This is probably the most self-evident and yet the ambiguous principle that allow the broadest interpretation. The "do no harm" principle exists in many health care codes of ethics (APA, AMA, and others), and NGOs that specialize in health care have also adopted it (Sheather et al., 2016). The World Medical Association (WMA, 2015, p. 120) has defined this principle as avoiding inflicting harm on patients and research subjects. This goal may not be easily attainable in the volatile context of GMH, where workers often resort to choosing between potentially harmful intervention—a choice that can be emotionally draining and even traumatizing for the providers (Cherepanov, 2017a).

In the 1965 science fiction novel *Monday Starts on Saturday*, the brothers Strugatsky (1965/2005) describe the imaginary Scientific Research Institute of Sorcery and Wizardry. This institute is populated by recognizable mythological personages who work there as regular researchers. In fact, this novel in a witty way describes the daily routine of a research institute where everyone is a little bit of a magician. Among others, there is an employee called Odin, whose name in Scandinavian mythology means "the ruler of gods." When the new IT director inquiries about his job responsibilities, he is told that Odin is so powerful that he can do anything. The only limitation is that he must not harm anybody by his actions. As a result, he gets paid for doing nothing (Figure 7.1).

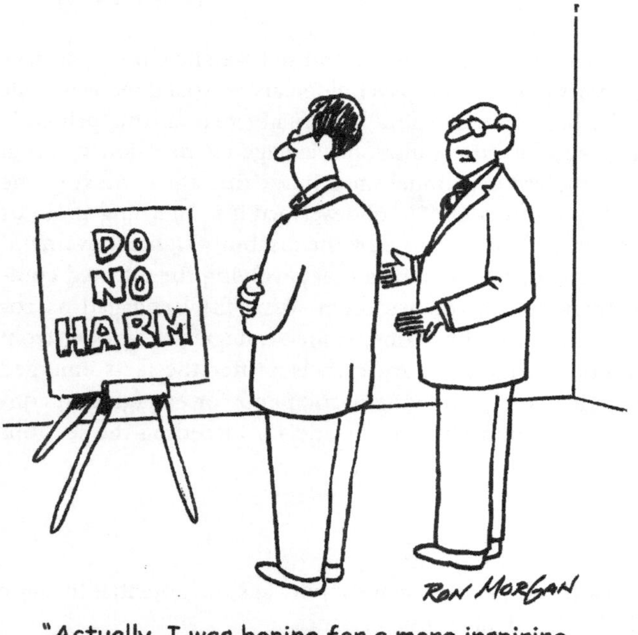

Figure 7.1 "Actually, I Was Hoping for a More Inspiring Mission Statement" (Cartoon by Ron Morgan, used with permission)

Building on Available Resources and Capacities

> All affected groups and individuals have assets or resources that support mental health recovery and psychosocial well-being.
>
> (IASC, 2007, p. 11)

This principle recognizes survivors' resilience and strength in the face of adversity and cautions against fostering dependence. Flannery and Everly (2000) described how the assumption that individuals have resources for recovery has been a ground principle for all crisis intervention modalities, such as psychological first aid, critical incident debriefing and disaster mental health. According to Flannery and Everly (2000), helping affected populations to recover and to become independent and self-reliant is achieved by actively facilitating problem solving, assisting in the development of appropriate strategies for addressing their concerns, and in helping to put those strategies into action. This suggests that in a crisis, the role of provider is not to "fix" problems but rather to identify and build upon existing strengths and resources.

A similar presumption lies in the foundation of the Community-Based Psychological Recovery in Complex Emergency (CBPR) model (Cherepanov, 2015a, 2016), which suggests strategies for engaging the affected community in recovery efforts. This approach aims at maximizing the sustainability of recovery through capacity building, empowerment, and training of local providers. It is also proposed that in situations of daily stresses and uncertainty, people can draw their strength not from hopes for the future (which can be rather uncertain) but rather from past survival experiences, as happened in the wake of the Chernobyl disaster (Cherepanov, 2011; Pearson & Cherepanov, 2012).

Integrated Support Systems

> Activities and programming should be integrated as far as possible. The proliferation of standalone services can create a highly fragmented care system.
>
> (IASC, 2007, p. 11)

The historical experience of humanitarian relief demonstrated the high price that the humanitarian community and its beneficiaries can pay for uncoordinated standalone services. Such fragmentation undermines the integrity and efficiency of aid, resulting in duplication of services and inefficient use of resources. As the MH and psychosocial module progresses toward integration into humanitarian action, the coordination of multidisciplinary efforts depends not only on the consistency of approaches but also on the consistency of methods. This means that GMH methods and tools must be compatible with the methods and agendas coming from different paradigms, an example of which would be the integrated MH and medical intervention for HIV and associated depression. If the integrated supports are not exercised, the opposite scenario (which I have observed on numerous occasions) would be if the medical and MH providers approach the treatment of HIV and depression separately, in different compounds, without even communicating to each other. These examples expose the danger of professional self-centeredness and indicate that in GMH the professionals need to work collaboratively on the goals shared by multidisciplinary actors.

In spite of all the progress toward establishing a comprehensive and consistent system of services, GMH still has a long way to go, and there seem to be several factors complicating this process:

1. Self-centeredness of the MH profession, which historically has struggled to emancipate itself from proxy disciplines, and where working as a part of multidisciplinary teams is a recent innovation.

   Way too often, I have observed MH providers in the field who felt they were the only ones who could help the survivors and conducted their work without any coordination or even communication with other multidisciplinary services on the ground.
2. Internal fragmentation and methodological differences within MH where the major approaches historically were developed based on exclusive paradigms: psychoanalysis, cognitive-behavioral therapy, expressive arts therapy, thought field therapy, and others.

   In this way, a psychoanalyst may have a very different understanding of a problem from a cognitive-behavior practitioner, and their proposed solutions may not be compatible or may even contradict each other. So much for teamwork!
3. Naïve narcissism of MH providers believing that the method they practice is the only one viable tool that universally works.

   I have also observed the negative impact of the rigidity in some approaches (I call it "virgin approaches," that preserve their purity and do not allow any modifications or inclusion of elements from other approaches) stemming from siloed paradigms in MH where different providers fail to adjust their methods to the realities of the situation or the clients' needs.

Multilayered Supports

> In emergencies, people are affected in different ways and require different kinds of supports. A key to organizing mental health and psychosocial support is to develop a layered system of complementary supports that meet the needs of different groups. All layers are important and should ideally be implemented concurrently.
>
> (IASC, 2007, p. 11)

This principle emphasizes the role of GMH as an integrated part of humanitarian action: We cannot do it alone, and the effectiveness of our work depends on complementary and collaborative efforts. This being said, a systematic review of MH and psychosocial support interventions targeting survivors of sexual and gender-based violence in conflict settings could not determine whether a comprehensive approach was effectively better than a targeted approach, possibly due to methodological flaws (Tol et al., 2013). The study concluded that more focused research efforts were needed to make this determination. Another "gray area" in implementing this guideline is supporting those who cannot benefit from complementary supports, e.g. cannot count on community or family supports, like survivors of gender-based violence or Ebola. The examples from the recent Ebola epidemics demonstrated how MSF psychosocial providers can be effective in providing standalone services against the IASC recommendations, and how they can individually support individuals who have become pariahs in their community (Rey, 2014).

7.3 Exercise: Using Operational Guidance for Designing Ethical Interventions

This exercise provides the opportunity to practice using operational guidance in designing ethical MH and psychosocial interventions. The goal is to recognize the ethical challenges in the interventions described in the vignettes and to change those interventions so that they are consistent with both the aspirational values and operational principles.

Instructions

Read the proposal for a MH intervention. Discuss the following points.

1. What is thought to be the intent or goal of the intervention?
2. What could be the unintended consequences?
3. What guideline or humanitarian value does it potentially challenge?
4. Make recommendations for revisions to these interventions so they are effective and ethical.

Example

An international NGO sponsors a summer camp for children from the affected region.

1. The intent of this intervention is to provide a safe and therapeutic space for children where they could begin a healing process.
2. The unintended consequences are that the selected children may not be those who need it the most. Instead, the local administration might object to the camp unless their own children and the children of their relatives are part of the program. In addition, there may be other children who want to participate and are eligible but the program cannot accommodate

them due to limited capacity. Another concern may be that the children may have difficulties readjusting to their routine life full of hardship and adversities.

3. This intervention challenges the "do no harm" principle. If poorly planned, this intervention can put participants and providers at risk because it may expose participants and make them targets for those who weren't able to take part.
4. Engaging the community, making the selection process transparent, and making the plans for reentry and aftercare supports key components would allow this program to be successful, ethical, and beneficial for the involved children. Additionally, the selection of the participants must be impartial and just, and appear as such to the community.

Practice Scenarios

1. A professor along with students travel to the affected region as part of the study. There, students under supervision learn how to provide trauma counseling.
2. A MH worker plans to travel to the affected area to train local providers in evidence-based exposure therapy.
3. A MH worker is interested in creating a stand-alone program to treat rape victims.
4. A prescriber creates a fund to supply psychotropic medications to disaster survivors.
5. An academic team travels to the affected area to perform an assessment related to the area of their research interest. They plan to publish data on symptom prevalence in a scientific journal, which will advance their career.
6. A MH provider wants to sponsor education for several children.
7. A MH provider brings to the affected region T-shirts with an empowering message to distribute among LGBTQ clients.
8. A MH provider who works with survivors of gender-based violence considers collaboration with local law enforcement to hold perpetrators accountable.

   Additional consideration:
   - What if this involves the disclosure of the victims' identity?
   - What if the governmental authorities are known to have been involved in violations of human rights and are siding up with the perpetrators?
9. A child reveals to a MH provider that she is being physically and sexually abused at home. The provider wants to assure safety for this child by notifying the local authorities.

CHAPTER 8

Ethical Dilemmas: Damned If You Do and Damned If You Don't

8.1 Ethical Dilemmas in Global Mental Health

Definition of an Ethical Dilemma

Behnke (2005) defined an ethical dilemma as a complex situation that involves an apparent mental conflict between moral imperatives in which to obey one would result in transgressing another. In the professional setting, these dilemmas create particular challenges because any compromise of professional standards or abandonment of any of the core values may not be acceptable. It is proposed that these dilemmas with no "either-or" solutions represent a false dichotomy that reflects the underlying conflict of paradigms. I also argue that when it is impossible to decide what values are "more valuable," placing conflicting values within a larger context removes this false opposition. For example, we cannot say which moral value "is more moral" or what professional value "is more professional" outside of a very specific context.

Let us examine this construct using the simple dilemma when we have to choose what color is better, white or black. Obviously, this dilemma is too abstract and cannot have a solution outside of the context. But we can negotiate it by using one of these strategies: (a) looking at the ideal design in the house and checking the overall consistency with other colors that are being used; (b) identifying where and for what purpose the colors will be used, and which color better serves this specific goal; or (c) establishing whether we are making this decision emotionally (e.g. which one has sentimental value), practically (e.g. which paint is cheaper and easier to maintain), or morally (e.g. some colors carry symbolic significance in certain contexts, like during a wedding or a funeral, for example).

Similarly, it is proposed that the strategies to approaching the intractable conflict of values can include: (a) establishing the contextual relevance of competing multidisciplinary agendas within a broader context of humanitarian work, (b) establishing priority of professional values based on accountability or determining the best use of resources, or (c) exerting self-awareness in navigating moral conundrums. These strategies as they apply to GMH will be discussed further, and case examples are provided at the end of the chapter.

In ethical dilemmas, the conflicting values can be multidisciplinary, professional, or moral. This chapter examines approaches to negotiating different dilemmas where both of the conflicting values belong to the same level, e.g. conflict between professional–professional or between moral–moral values. Cross-level dilemmas (e.g. conflict between professional and moral values) fall outside of the scope of this work.

8.2 Reconciling Multidisciplinary Agendas: Engaging a Higher Level of Values

The Conflicts of Multidisciplinary Agendas

An example of the competing multidisciplinary agenda can be a situation when an NGO with limited resources has to choose between prioritizing education (i.e. establishing a school for adults and children) or health care (i.e. setting up an outpatient clinic). In an ideal world, these complementary agendas should not conflict and can and should be implemented concurrently. In reality, however, the allocation of the resources can present a daunting task. Both modules seem equally important and the decision that brings most benefits would depend on the context. During the health crisis, health care becomes a humanitarian priority because it saves more lives, and education comes to the forefront in the context of long-term agenda. "As much as my duty is to advocate for the priority of MH services, with the right amount of humility, I unconditionally yield the right of way to sanitation" (E. Cherepanov, personal communication, November 18, 2016).

Clarinval and Biller-Andorno (2014) argue that competing multidisciplinary agendas are inevitable in humanitarian action. According to the authors, the humanitarian action is based on multifarious sets of values explicitly or implicitly held by humanitarian actors, organizations, and donors. Certain values represent the substantive views of the organization, such as impartiality, independence, or religious beliefs. Other values prioritize procedure, such as accountability, transparency, and needs-based approaches. Some values seem more universal, like humanitarian values, while others are profession specific. Wilson (2009) believed that cross-sectoral conflicts of values are caused by fragmented silos of policy-making and viewed values reconciliation as a contribution to the defragmentation of humanitarian efforts. Rokhideh (2017) described the detrimental impact of siloed multidisciplinary interventions in post-conflict northern Uganda. She concluded that by approaching multidisciplinary planning as a component of a larger agenda, such as peace building, could lead to the development of a shared cross-sectorial vision making possible a holistic approach, which she understood as a multi-sectional and multi-layered integrated approach.

To promote cohesiveness in multidisciplinary interventions, the Sphere Project (2011) outlined an overreaching framework for multidisciplinary interactions and proposed the concept of the humanitarian charter and minimum standards. However, conflicting multidisciplinary agendas still remain one of the biggest challenges for humanitarians who are working to advance a common goal via their own professional mission. When different agendas compete, this puts further pressure on aid workers to navigate conflicting humanitarian priorities with integrity and professionalism.

Navigating Competing Multidisciplinary Agendas

The professional literature describes several approaches to reconciling conflicts between multidisciplinary agendas: the process-oriented approach, placing values into the broader context, and engaging the higher level of values.

Five-Step Process for Resolving Intractable Dilemmas

Pearce and Littlejohn (1997, p. 20) examined complex multidisciplinary conflicts where multiple agendas and systems of values collided to create intractable dilemmas. They suggested a five-step process:

1. Uncover the conflict of values.
2. Develop categories to compare incommensurable differences.
3. Seek to explore rather than convince.
4. Assess the strengths and weaknesses of both worldviews.
5. Seek to reframe the conflict into more productive terms.

Placing Values Into the Broader Context

Another way to approach this conflict is to resolve the false opposition by placing the dilemmas into a larger context. Rokhideh (2017) used peace-building activities to examine the idea that the conflict between multidisciplinary values may be "false paradigmatic oppositions" that get resolved once they are placed by introducing a broad shared framework—the peace-building efforts, in her case.

Engaging a Higher Level of Values

The approach proposed here suggests that when multidisciplinary values collide, the decision can be made by engaging higher levels of values, such as the universal humanitarian values that are shared by all humanitarian actors and serve as a broader frame of reference for conflicting cross-sectional and multidisciplinary agendas. Engaging higher or meta levels of values means that, when a dilemma cannot be resolved on one level, a professional can appeal to the humanitarian ideals, which remind us of what we all are doing and why (Cherepanov, 2017a). Previously I argued that for a GMH professional (as well as for any other professional actors), different values may carry different priorities based on their contextual relevance (Cherepanov, 2017a). The engagement of humanitarian principles, which are the meta-level values for humanitarian actors, helps to

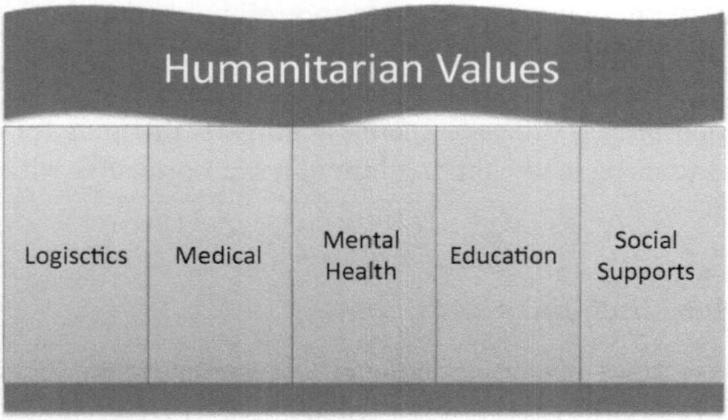

Figure 8.1 Engagement of Humanitarian Values to Reconcile the Conflicting Multidisciplinary Agenda

initiate a dialog and establish productive collaborations between representatives of different disciplines and sections. It is important to note that prioritizing professional values does not equate to prioritizing MH needs, but rather reflects establishing a primacy of values for professional decision-making.

Figure 8.1 illustrates the overarching role of humanitarian ideals, which provide a shared context and common ground for multidisciplinary humanitarian actors.

8.3 Managing Professional Dilemmas: Establishing Accountability

It may be particularly problematic to choose between equally essential professional values for the providers who take pride in their professional integrity. In a documentary Orbinski (2008) described this impossible dilemma as "racing against time with limited resources, when relief workers make split-second decisions: who gets treatment; who gets food; who lives; who dies."

The publications by ethicists from different backgrounds (Pearce & Littlejohn, 1997; Reisch & Lowe, 2008; Wilson, 2009) and the models mentioned in often anonymous pages of websites such as Ask.com, Wiki Answers, PowerpointShare, or Wikipedia, identify several approaches to reasoning the professional dilemmas. They are: pre-determined priorities and protocol-based approaches, employing different levels of references in decision-making, and establishing accountability.

Different Approaches to Resolving Professional Dilemmas

Predetermined Priorities

The normative and protocol-based approaches to professional dilemmas set the expectations about the norms and determine priorities or the protocols for decision-making. The pre-defined norms and procedures can improve the transparency, accountability, and quality of decisions (Kidder, 1995/2005; Li et al., 2016;

Reisch & Lowe, 2008). Loewenberg and Dolgoff (1992, p. 63) suggested that, while all values are important for a professional, some are objectively more important than others. They proposed the Ethical Rules Screen model, which ranks values based on their significance in decision-making. Their hierarchy of values hierarchy consists of seven basic values and principles ranked in descending order:

1. Protection of life.
2. Equality and inequality.
3. Autonomy and freedom.
4. Least harm.
5. Quality of life.
6. Privacy and confidentiality.
7. Truthfulness and full disclosure.

This model helps to map the priorities in decision-making; however, it leaves out the rationale for this particular order. While the primacy of "protection of life" is indisputable, the position of the remaining values appear arbitrary: why is "equality" ranked as a higher priority than "autonomy and freedom" and "least harm"? Are there any circumstances when these priorities can change?

In another example, the Josephson Institute of Ethics (2002) offered the seven-step protocol structuring decision-making, which is based on the assumption that making ethical choices requires the ability to make distinctions between competing options.

1. *Stop and think.* This provides several benefits. It prevents rash decisions, prepares us for more thoughtful discernment, and can allow us to mobilize our discipline.
2. *Clarify goals.* Before you choose, clarify your short-term and long-term aims. Determine which of your many wants and "don't wants" affected by the decision are the most important. The big danger is that decisions that fulfill immediate wants and needs can prevent the achievement of our more important life goals.
3. *Determine facts.* Be sure you have adequate information to support an intelligent choice. To determine the facts, first resolve what you know, then what you need to know. Be prepared for additional information and to verify assumptions and other uncertain information. In addition:
   - Consider the reliability and credibility of the people providing the facts.
   - Consider the basis of the supposed facts. If the person giving you the information says he or she personally heard or saw something, evaluate that person in terms of honesty, accuracy, and memory.
4. *Develop options.* Once you know what you want to achieve and have made your best judgment as to the relevant facts, make a list of actions you can take to accomplish your goals. If it's an especially important decision, talk to someone

you trust to gain a broader perspective and think of new choices. If you can think of only one or two choices, you're probably not thinking hard enough.

5. *Consider consequences.* Filter your choices to determine if any of your options will violate any core ethical values, and then eliminate any unethical options. Identify who will be affected by the decision and how the decision is likely to affect them.
6. *Choose.* Make a decision. If the choice is not immediately clear, try the following:
   - Talk to people whose judgment you respect.
   - Think of a person of strong character that you know or know of, and ask yourself what they would do in your situation.
   - If everyone found out about your decision, would you be proud and comfortable?
   - Follow the golden rule: treat others the way you want to be treated, and keep your promises.
7. *Monitor and modify.* Ethical decision makers monitor the effects of their choices. If they are not producing the intended results, or are causing additional unintended and undesirable results, they reassess the situation and make new decisions.

Levels of Reference in Decision-Making

In an original approach, Clarinval and Biller-Andorno (2014) used the inherent contradiction between population-focused public health and individual-focused clinical frameworks to suggest that attributing values to the different levels of decision-making, namely at the macro, meso, and micro level (respectfully headquarters, country/region, and delegate/beneficiary levels), would allow for establishing different levels of reference or accountability.

Establishing Accountability

In opposition to the "one size fits all" normative approaches, a values-based framework prioritizes solutions that are consistent with humanitarian values, minimize harm, and establish professional accountability. At the same time, having a frame of a reference that is broad and flexible enough to encompass complex dilemmas and moral uncertainties comes with a price. Not having the pre-determined solutions places more responsibility on the professional to make informed choices and elevates the role of professional judgment, competency, and personal integrity in the decision-making process. It is proposed that humanitarian accountability or who we are primarily accountable to (e.g. organization, profession, the populations we serve), can help to determine which intervention is the most consistent with the demands of situation and the provider's role.

Figure 8.2 illustrates the role of professional accountability in navigating the dilemma where a MHPSS provider should decide whether to administer the focus

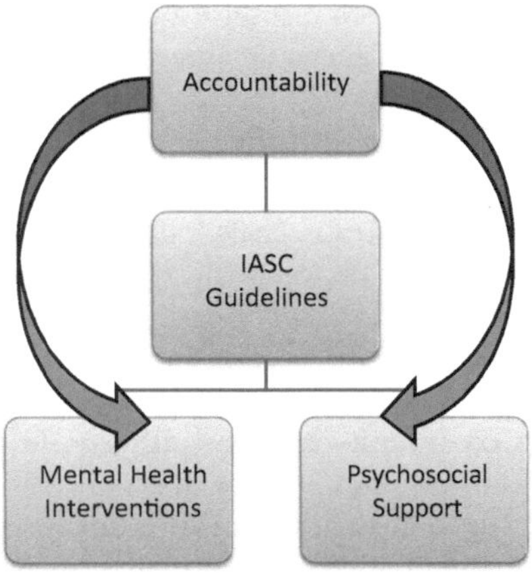

Figure 8.2 Accountability in Professional Dilemmas

interventions for people with a higher level of MH needs or to use resources for strengthening community and family supports. According to the IASC pyramid of MH and psychosocial supports, both modalities are complementary and must be implemented concurrently. If they conflict, the decision is made based on accountability, which establishes the primary point of reference.

Below are common professional dilemmas in GMH followed by discussions illustrating the role of accountability in the decision-making.

Examples

1. To Treat, Support, or Prevent?

Sometimes providers have to choose whether to focus their interventions and allocate resources on treating persons in need or invest in organizing community supports and focusing on community development and prevention. In such cases, referring to the IASC guidelines allows designing interventions as complementary, where, for example, the community-wide intervention can focus on destigmatizing mental illnesses and establishing mutual supports.

2. To Respond or to Develop?

Having to choose between the response and the development modes of intervention is a familiar dilemma for humanitarian action. This basically means having to choose between attending to immediate or long-term needs. These conflicting priorities reflect the profound difference in professional priorities that affect operations and ignite competition for resources. In this case, the universal value of humanitarian accountability allows us to better negotiate and reconcile priorities. Within the accountability framework, the discourse translates into the planning of the interventions in such a way that they incorporate both response and developmental modes, which, in the given example, can mean engaging and training the local providers while providing relief.

3. To Quarantine or Not to Quarantine?

The infamous methodological conflict between clinical versus public health approaches translates among others into the conflict between the rights of an individual and the rights of the community. This situation can be easily imagined in the case of an infectious disease outbreak. Focusing on treating individuals at home increases the risk of spreading the infection, while involuntary quarantine aims at containing the infection but hinders community trust, resulting in less reporting about new cases. What to choose? The "either-or" approach is not really applicable here, as both options appear equally to come with a price. This dilemma opens up the opportunity to discuss a wide range of approaches: weighing what results in lesser mortality and morbidity, social and psychological fallout of the mandatory isolation of those who are infected, building trust with the community, providing health education about the symptoms and the importance of getting treatment, fighting rumors and conspiracy theories, and providing psychological support to the affected families. The introjection of accountability allows determining to whom the providers are primarily accountable in their professional capacity, individual patients, community, families, and what would be most beneficial in this role.

8.4 Negotiating Moral Conundrums: A Heuristic Approach

A moral dilemma is understood as a conflict between two mutually exclusive moral imperatives, neither of which can be unambiguously accepted or preferred. The main feature of moral conundrums is that no matter what the decision is, it carries the potential to inflict a moral injury. Moral conundrums are unsolvable by definition, but reflecting on how decisions are made can help to choose the option with the greatest contextual relevance.

Perhaps the most widely discussed impossible moral dilemma is the one depicted in the movie *Sophie's Choice*, based on the William Styron novel (1979). In the movie, Sophie and her two children are in a Nazi concentration camp. A guard tells Sophie that one of her children will be allowed to live and one will be killed. But it is Sophie who must decide which child will be killed. Sophie can prevent the death of either of her children, but only by condemning the other; if she chooses neither, then both will be killed. Of her two children, Sophie chooses to sacrifice her 7-year-old daughter, Eva, in a heart-wrenching decision that leaves her with a profound feeling of guilt that she isn't able to overcome, leading her to a deep depression and self-destructive alcoholism.

Having to make a morally difficult decision puts tremendous moral pressure on professionals who may find themselves in the position of having to choose whether rescuing one life is more important than putting the larger community at risk;

or how to leave behind local staff and abandon clients during evacuation. Even when professionals know what the right thing to do is, their deep-seated moral or spiritual convictions may tell them otherwise, creating an irreconcilable dissonance that can be very traumatizing. I have known aid workers for whom mere exposure to the existential abyss of a moral conundrum has become a profoundly traumatizing experience and who have remained haunted by the memories and nightmares many years later. They have consistently named the post-deployment debriefings, peer supports, and individual therapy as the most helpful tools for sorting out conflicting feelings.

The *Oxford Dictionary* defines heuristics as "proceeding to a solution ... by rules that are only loosely defined" (Oxford Online Dictionary, s.v. "heuristic"). Where finding an optimal solution to a moral conundrum is impossible or impractical, the heuristic approach can be used to speed up the process of finding a satisfactory solution, or serve as a shortcut. This approach refers to a mental shortcut, which does not guarantee to be optimal or perfect, but sufficient for the immediate goals. In practical terms, the heuristic approach to reasoning moral dilemmas could mean establishing differences between emotional, moral, rational, and professional levels or modes of decision-making, and making the informed choice about the level that is most appropriate to the situation.

Schwarz (2000) argued that decisions can differ depending on whether they are made emotionally or rationally. If we are to extrapolate this approach to reasoning our way through moral dilemmas, it is possible to infer that GMH decisions can be made on different levels:

- *emotional level* or what our feelings or instincts tell us about what is the right thing to do;
- *moral level* or decisions based on personal, spiritual, or existential convictions and beliefs that give us the sense that we are worthy human beings;
- *rational level* or decisions arrived at by comparing different outcomes, like determining what brings the greater benefit and inflicts lesser harm;
- *professional level* or adherence to professional standards.

Figure 8.3 illustrates the relationships between different levels of reasoning. Recognizing how feelings, personal values, and beliefs impact our choices and moving toward the professional level of decision-making can be both productive and therapeutic as it reduces emotional investment and helps us make informed and professional decisions based on the analysis of available choices and their situational relevance.

Example

A MH professional works as part of a multidisciplinary team to assist with post-disaster recovery. The community struggles with shortages of food and water,

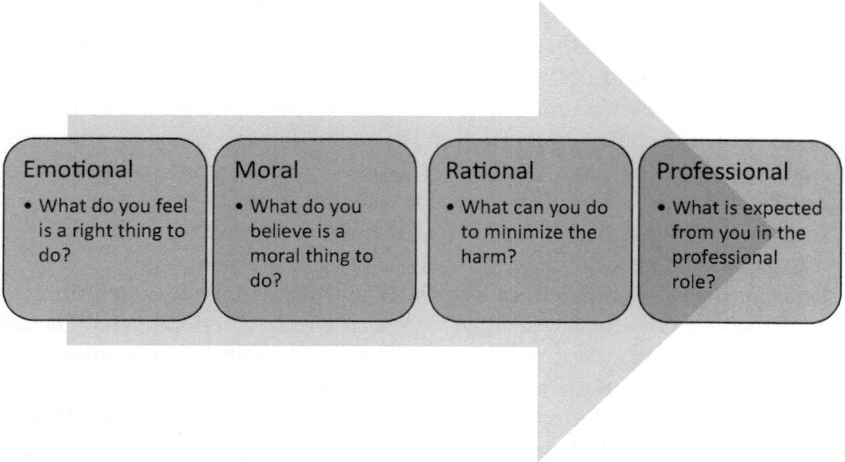

Figure 8.3 Reasoning Moral Dilemmas

violence, and severe trauma. Hungry children beg for food. A provider feels that he/she is unable to eat when children are hungry and gives his/her own food to them.

Discussion

This example contains several moral dilemmas at once. On an emotional level, the provider's response is understandable: we are hardwired to viscerally respond to suffering in children, and hungry children are always a powerful trigger. The moral or spiritual reasoning also supports the provider's choice, as from a moral standpoint we are expected to share with those in need.

When making decisions from a professional role, a provider can weigh different options and compare outcomes, seek guidance from supervisors, and advocate for increases in nutritional aid in the community. The questions to ask yourself in this situation may be:

- How effective can the provider who does not eat be? Will he/she be able to do the work?
- Obviously, there will not be enough food to share with all children in need. How will the provider decide who needs food more?
- What's more beneficial for the community: to feed several children or to help more children by being able to continue working?
- In a situation where there is a competition for resources, will sharing a meal with some children put them at risk for retaliation?

Needless to say, exposure to moral dilemmas can be extremely emotionally draining and traumatizing, and psychological supports are important tools for coping with survivor guilt and conflicting feelings.

8.5 Exercise: Unsolvable Conundrums—What Would You Do?

Instructions

1. Read the moral dilemmas.
2. Negotiate the conundrum on the emotional, moral, cognitive, and professional levels.
3. Compare outcomes and brainstorm possible personal and professional implications at each level.

Example: A Paraphrase of One of the Fundamental Moral Conundrums

A Boat With Six People Is Sinking … Among Them

A child
A Nobel Prize laureate
A homeless alcoholic
A disabled person
A mother of three
A fellow humanitarian worker

You can rescue only one person … Who will you rescue?

Discussion

While *emotionally* we may be compelled to rescue a child, from the *moral* standpoint, there may be an inclination to rescue either a disabled person or the child. *Rationally*, saving the mother of three or the Nobel Prize laureate may have the biggest impact on the well-being of the most people. The alternative rational solution may be this: we cannot decide whose life is more valuable and every person must have an equal chance to survive. Thus, everyone must have an equal chance to be rescued. In this case, the rescuer, for instance, can try for the one who is closest.

The *professional* solution here seems to be the least counterintuitive: in the field, it is expected that all efforts will be made to rescue a fellow aid worker first. This decision is based on the bigger picture: if an expatriate is hurt, the international political repercussions may be greater and result in the termination of aid delivery that can put many more people in danger. This rationale, however, doesn't sit well morally, and should a similar situation happen in the field, it must be followed up with a debriefing and mobilization of psychological supports.

Practice Case Scenarios for Reasoning Moral Dilemmas. What Would You Do?

1. A terminally ill 3-year-old child has several days to live if he receives oxygen. The family requests that the child be taken home to die surrounded by his loving family, but the treating provider is against it because the boy will not survive travel. How can you facilitate the discussion aiming at finding the most appropriate solution to this moral dilemma?

   What if this child is a suspected to have communicable disease?
2. At a medical compound treating very sick people in a refugee camp, a crowd of angry people is chasing a man. He approaches the medical compound and begs for refuge.

   What if a female victim of domestic violence asks you to hide her on the compound?
3. A children-focused organization delivers a limited supply of food for children to a remote area. The community leaders say that the food must first go to the elderly because they are more valuable members of the community. You are a respected MH provider in the community and have opportunity to affect the decision.
4. You work with survivors in the affected area. Violence breaks out and threatens the aid workers. The site director orders an evacuation:
   a. The survivors are scared and ask you not to leave them in danger.
   b. The car is sent to evacuate the expatriates. At the last moment, there is a family of the local aid worker with little children who beg you to help them.

CHAPTER 9

Ethically Questionable Practices

Carl Jung wrote, "until you make the unconscious conscious, it will direct your life and you will call it fate" (Jung, 1979, p.126). This means that we can only manage the issues we are aware of, and this chapter deconstructs some of the most common cognitive alterations in GMH that implicitly or explicitly affect professional judgment and integrity of care. The vulnerability of a traumatized population is the very reason why trauma work mandates professional trustworthiness and the highest ethical standards in relating to survivors. At the same time, trauma work carries the potential to trigger providers' own traumatic experiences and actualize their unmet needs. Addressing self-awareness in the training or supervisory context allows GMH professionals to more effectively address cognitive distortions such as countertransference, biases, and privileges, and raise awareness about preconceived notions and stereotypes.

9.1 Countertransference: A Threat to Professional and Personal Boundaries

Countertransference occurs when a client's experience triggers providers' traumatic memories and elicits personal emotional reactions that can compromise the provider's ability to respond to the client's needs. In *The Future Prospects of Psycho-Analytic Therapy*, Sigmund Freud in 1910 defined countertransference as being "a result of the patient's influence on [the physician's] unconscious feelings" (cited in Laplanche & Pontalis, 1988, pp. 92–93). Braak (2002) associated the providers' countertransference with traumatized clients' unmet needs for safety, trust, personal power, or control, and esteem and intimacy. This triggers strong emotions in providers who may share similar needs. Williams (2012) went on to identify countertransference as the biggest threat to professional and personal boundaries in those who work with severe trauma because the other people's trauma may trigger providers' personal experiences and cause them to act in a way that they would not have done otherwise. When these boundaries are blurred, any aspect of what is allowed in the therapeutic relationship can appear ambiguous. Such ambiguity is often experienced as an intrusion and leaves clients feeling unsafe. Pain from a violation of boundaries may come as a delayed reaction, and the violation itself may not even be recognized or felt until later harmful consequences emerge or become evident. Williams (2012) asserted the crucial role of self-awareness for traumatologists in recognizing countertransference and managing unconscious cognitive distortions because they present a threat to professional boundaries and integrity of care and lead to burnout. According to Williams, countertransference must be treated with full seriousness and can be best addressed by means of self-care, therapy, and supervision.

The impact of countertransference in MH work has been studied comparatively well in the context of the therapeutic alliance and helpers' burnout (e.g. Rothschild, 2006). Here we will focus on "victim blaming," "rescue fantasy," "survivor guilt," and other phenomena that are associated with countertransference in GMH work.

Anna Freud (1946) explained "victim blaming" or identification with the aggressor as a primitive defense mechanism, which involves projection of guilt and anger toward the victim of aggression. Another account was offered by Lerner and Miller (1978), who linked victim blaming to "a just world" fallacy, or the belief that "bad things do not happen to good people." The belief that people deserve what happens to them stems from the basic human need for predictability. Otherwise, the world is perceived as unsafe and unpredictable, where anything can happen to anyone.

Victim blaming comes in many forms and shapes. It can present as anger toward survivors for historically contributing to the conflict, or for not doing enough to help themselves, or misusing the aid, or even for not showing enough appreciation for the help provided to them. In my experience, this anger can also be shaped as a belief that survivors overly dramatize their suffering and exaggerate their needs to elicit pity.

> After the devastating Spitak earthquake in Armenia in 1988, the aid workers who flocked into the area expressed anger toward local men who were waiting for help instead of trying to organize their own recovery missions. Only education about the phases of the psychological response to catastrophic events followed by mass casualties helped rescue workers to accept that they must rely on their own resources because survivors may have been demoralized by the scale of the disaster. As more time passed, more locals joined the efforts.
>
> (E. Cherepanov, personal communication, July 14, 1990)

"Rescuer fantasy" is a subconscious belief or fantasy centering on rescue, or a belief that one must rescue or save another person from something bad, posited as a motive for certain actions or choices (Oxford Online Dictionary, s.v. "rescuer fantasy"). When acting upon a rescuer fantasy, a provider feels that he/she is alone charged with the rescue mission and saving human lives. A rescuer fantasy, or "the superman complex," comes with an illusion of omnipotence and irreplaceability and inflated perception of one's own role. It also is associated with perceiving other people as incapable of making informed decisions. Overestimating an individual

Table 9.1 The Belief System of the White Savior Industrial Complex (Twitter Thread by Teju Cole (@tejucole, 2012))

1	From Sachs to Kristof to Invisible Children to TED, the fastest growth industry in the US is the White Savior Industrial Complex.
2	The White savior supports brutal policies in the morning, founds charities in the afternoon, and receives awards in the evening.
3	The banality of evil transmutes into the banality of sentimentality. The world is nothing but a problem to be solved by enthusiasm.
4	This world exists simply to satisfy the needs—including, importantly, the sentimental needs—of White people and Oprah.
5	The White Savior Industrial Complex is not about justice. It is about having a big emotional experience that validates privilege.
6	Feverish worry over that awful African warlord. But close to 1.5 million Iraqis died from an American war of choice. Worry about that.
7	I deeply respect American sentimentality, the way one respects a wounded hippo. You must keep an eye on it, for you know it is deadly.

provider's role in GMH contradicts the principle of collaborative effort, which is the ground principle of humanitarian action.

The "White savior" complex refers to a White person who acts to help non-White people in a self-serving manner. The role is considered a modern-day version of what is expressed in the poem, "The White Man's Burden," by Rudyard Kipling (1899/1997) (see more in the description of the "missionary bias" below). The term has been associated with Africa, and certain characters in films and television that have been critiqued as White savior figures. Writer Teju Cole (2012) combined the term with "industrial complex" (derived from the military-industrial complex and similarly applied elsewhere) to coin the term "White Savior Industrial Complex." Cole used Twitter to formulate a hilarious belief system of self-absorbed Westerners who travel to Third World countries and make the entire affair an exercise in self-congratulatory sacrifice. The belief system of the White Savior Industrial Complex is summarized in Table 9.1

"Survivor guilt" was first recognized during the 1960s as part of "survivor's syndrome," also called "concentration camp survivor's syndrome" (Krell & Eitinger, 1985). It is understood as a mental condition that occurs when a person perceives that they have somehow done wrong by surviving a traumatic event when others did not. Sufferers sometimes blame themselves for the death and suffering of others or experience irrational guilt for being alive and well while others are not. Katz and Segall (1976), described a variation of survivor guilt—so-called "White guilt"—which they defined as the individual or collective guilt felt by some White people for harm resulting from racist treatment of ethnic minorities. And indeed, some expatriates have shared with me feelings of guilt toward multicultural clientele and national staff because they are White and haven't been subjected to racism or because they come from more well-off countries.

Survivor guilt in fieldworkers can be particularly dangerous when it triggers self-destructive inclinations or self-neglect when a provider feels that their life does not matter or they do not deserve to be happy or even to live when others suffer or die. This altered perception hinders the compliance with the safety imperative.

9.2 Cognitive Biases, Power Differential, and Privileges

Biases

Biases are the prejudices or preconceived notions in favor of or against one person or group (Oxford Online Dictionary, s.v. "bias"). Biases distort information interpretation and affect decisions and human behavior. Not all biases are negative, and positive biases may be the very reasons why some MH providers are interested in working with certain populations or cultures. The list of biases can be very long, and here I review only those relevant to GMH work.

"Missionary" or "colonizatory" bias initially referred to Rudyard Kipling's portrayals of Indian characters that generally supported the view that colonized people were incapable of surviving without the help of Europeans (Kipling, 1899/1997). This bias received its name from China Mills (2013), author of the book *Decolonizing Global Mental Health: The Psychiatrization of the Majority World*, who claimed that GMH is a form of colonialism that comes from within and from outside, swallowed in the form of a pill. Later, its meaning broadened and now it refers to a paternalistic and condescending attitude toward non-Westerners, who are perceived as incapable and helpless, and who must be guided in making the right choices.

Lipsky (1987) introduced the similar "dominant culture" bias, understood as a form of internalized racism or the conscious or subconscious acceptance of the dominant society's racist views, stereotypes, and biases concerning other ethnic groups. This bias gives rise to patterns of thinking, feeling, and behaving that result in discriminating, minimizing, criticizing, finding fault, invalidating, and hating oneself for belonging to the dominant culture.

"Ethnocentric" bias is similar to "dominant culture" bias, and means, as Brewer (2015) described, the tendency to view the world through the lens of one's own culture. That is, when individuals tend to judge others' behaviors, customs, beliefs, and attitudes by their own cultural standards.

Privileges

The *Oxford English Dictionary* defines privilege as a special right, advantage, or immunity granted or available only to a particular person or group (Oxford Online Dictionary, s.v. "privilege"). Privilege stems from a power disbalance. If not recognized by a self-aware provider, biases and privileges can set the stage for cognitive distortions and the intentional or unintentional abuse of power and other ethically questionable practices. The inherent disbalance of power between a helper and beneficiary is an attribute of any helping relationship, but it gains a whole new meaning in GMH due to the extreme vulnerabilities and pressing needs of the affected populations. Next, I will examine such privileges, examples of which have been found in the literature, information space, or were drawn from my experience.

According to McIntosh (1990, p. 5), "White privileges" are when Whites enjoy advantages that non-Whites do not experience, which is "an invisible package of unearned assets." This includes cultural affirmations of one's own worth and importance based primarily on race. The concept of White privilege also implies the right to assume the universality of one's own experiences, marking others as different or "not-normal."

In the same book, McIntosh (1990) defined "gender privileges," arguing that for many coming from traditional cultures, having a male gender confers an undue advantage to a provider who then enjoys greater respect from clients and is perceived as more trustworthy than female providers.

There are additional privileges affecting the provider–client alliance, which are relevant to GMH work. These are informational, socioeconomic, and expert privileges.

A service provider with "informational privileges" is a holder of valuable knowledge about resources that the clientele has no access to. This provider also has the perceived power to choose what information to release and to whom.

"Socioeconomic privileges" refer to the perception that a provider has power due to their higher socioeconomic status.

"Expert privileges" reflect the belief that doctors and other professionals have special knowledge and expertise allowing them to make decisions and recommendations that must not be questioned.

Table 9.2 summarizes the cognitive distortions and misperceptions common in GMH work.

9.3 Ethically Questionable Practices and Medication Misuse

In GMH, ethically questionable practices carry very serious consequences and can tarnish the image of the profession, which means less lifesaving aid and higher risks for humanitarians. The following communications from Pittaway et al. (2010) offer a poignant description of the impact of ethically questionable research practices.

> You know many of the organizations came to the refugee camp and they see the refugees in many ways as the monkeys ... like a monkey in a cage ... and then they thought that if we show this monkey to ... the big countries of power like the EU [European Union], they will have a lot of money and it will benefit us [the nongovernment organizations] ... They documented things [stories] of the women that are oppressed, then when they get money they use some for the refugees but mostly they use for themselves.
>
> (Discussion with a men's refugee group, Thai–Burma border, in Pittaway et al., 2010, p. 321)

Table 9.2 Cognitive Biases in Global Mental Health

Cognitive Distortion	*Definition*	*Examples*	*Cause*
Countertransference	Mostly unconscious reactions to a patient that are determined by the provider's own life history	Excessive anger toward the client: "Rescue fantasy" "Survivor guilt" "White guilt"	Identification with the victim or perpetrator Belief in a just world
Biases	Prejudice in favor of or against one thing, person, or group compared with another, usually in a way considered to be unfair	"Colonial or missionary bias" "Host country bias" "Ethnocenric bias" "Expert's bias"	Cognitive stereotypes and prejudices influenced by societal or family norms
Privileges	Prerogative referring to a special advantage or right possessed by an individual or group	"White privileges" "Host country privileges" "Gender privileges" "Socioeconomic privileges" "Expert privileges"	Power differential

> When I go into a horrendous camp situation as a White researcher, the people are so desperate for any form of assistance they would agree to anything just on the off-chance that I might be able to assist. It makes asking for permission to interview them or take photographs a farce ... What does "informed consent" mean in an isolated refugee camp with security problems and no proper interpreters?
>
> (Pittaway et al., 2010, p. 320)

> They asked us to lead them to women who had been raped so they could record their stories. "Tell us what happened—how did you feel?" Women were so upset after the interviews, we did not know what to do. We never heard from them [the researchers] again—we decided then that we would never work with researchers again. They stole our stories. We can gather the stories ourselves from our own people—you can help [with training].
>
> (Discussion with a women's group, Thailand, in Pittaway et al., 2010, p. 326)

The unethical practices where there is an intentional and gross disregard for law and codes of ethics fall outside of the scope of our subject. Not all harm, however, is done intentionally or willfully, and there are ethically questionable practices that stem from compromised judgment or cognitive distortions. The following examples of such practices were reported in the literature, came from the providers and beneficiaries' reports, and were drawn from my experience.

Iatrogenic Practices

Even the best of intentions can inflict harm when the well-meaning providers do not recognize the potentially iatrogenic impact of their interventions. In their book *Helping the Helpers Not to Harm*, Caplan and Caplan (2001, p. 22) defined iatrogenic harm as damage induced as a byproduct of an intervention, by a service provider or caretaker of any type, or from a procedure or technique. It can also be harm caused by the caregiving system. The Croatian-Austrian philosopher Illich (1974, p. 12), an avid critic of the institutions of modern Western culture, defined the social and cultural impact of iatrogenesis at three levels:

> First, clinical iatrogenesis is the injury done to patients by ineffective, unsafe, and erroneous treatments.
>
> Second, social iatrogenesis refers to the medicalization of suffering in which medical professionals, pharmaceutical companies, and medical device companies have a vested interest in sponsoring sickness by creating unrealistic health demands that require more treatments or to treat non-diseases that are part of the normal human experience, such as age-related declines. In this way, aspects of medical practice and medical-associated industries can produce social harm in which society members ultimately become less healthy, excessively dependent on institutional care [...]
>
> And third, cultural iatrogenesis refers to the destruction of traditional ways of dealing with, and making sense of, death, suffering, and sickness. In this way, the medicalization of life leads to cultural harm as society members lose their autonomous coping skills.

The over diagnosis of MH conditions can easily rise to the level of psychological iatrogenesis. Summerfield (2013) went on to classify these interventions as a form of medical imperialism: people who respond "normally" to extreme life adversities are persuaded that they have mental disorders and are offered a solution through the use of psychotropic medications. Clark (2014), who shared these concerns, emphasized the increased risks for iatrogenic harm in a time of globalization of MH and questioned the universality of biomedical concepts across cultures, which has been strongly disputed by transcultural psychiatrists and anthropologists.

Distorting Professional Role

Exposure to extreme emotions and countertransference can make it difficult to maintain impartiality and professional boundaries. I personally am aware of one psychologist who worked with a population affected by ethnic conflict and who ended up joining the resistance. Even though he went on to become a national hero (his name and the name of the conflict are intentionally omitted), his ability to work within a professional capacity and provide psychological supports was severely compromised.

Inadequate Planning of Interventions

Inadequate planning is viewed here as an ethically questionable practice that can inflict harm, as opposed to simply being a professional issue. Rokhideh (2017) used data to provide a powerful example of the fallout of inadequately planned psychosocial interventions in northern Uganda that coincided with increased rates of suicide, increased domestic violence, and increased substance abuse. While the link between these developments may have other explanations, the data draw attention to the core questions about how we define and measure success against the "do no harm" imperative. Reported instances where beneficiaries were abandoned by providers, left without established continuity of care and community supports, and ended up being increasingly isolated, exposed, and vulnerable, have raised valid ethical concerns. The author diagnosed this problem as the failure to adjust interventions to the complex and changing realities of post-conflict setting. In addition, some of these problematic outcomes can be explained by the fragmented nature of interventions and funding, while others indicate a lack of consistency and intersectional coordination, which has long been recognized as a challenge for humanitarian action. The described dilemma brings us back to the question of whether it is ethical to administer helping interventions where it is difficult to evaluate their impact.

Contextual Inappropriateness or Lacking a "Sense of Stage"

The term "sense of stage," or contextual appropriateness, comes from psychodrama. It was originally described by the philosopher Hannah Arendt (1983, p. 92) as the interplay between *being and appearing*. She went on to argue that everything we do is meant to be perceived by somebody, a "spectator." To have "a sense of stage" means to be contextually appropriate and aware of how our actions may appear to this spectator. For example, some actions that are perfectly appropriate in some situations may appear inappropriate in others, or as we say now, to "have bad optics." For instance, wearing expensive jewelry is appropriate at a banquet or conference, but wearing them when doing fieldwork or helping the homeless may display a different connotation. The sense of stage or contextual appropriateness underscores the inherent power differential between actor and audience, professor and student, clinician and patient, and helper and those being helped. Due to the nature of such relationships, a person in a role of power needs to consider not only what is said or done but also how it can be perceived by those with less power.

We already mentioned how important it is that any interventions not only be just, but also appear as such. When someone is lacking a sense of stage, they can lose perspective of their professional role and display conduct that appears unethical even though it would not have been regarded this way in other circumstances. A good example of the importance of this perception is in charity work. Photographs taken in the field by Western volunteers can be judged differently based on the context in which the photographs are taken, to avoid connotation with painting themselves as saviors to needy people in low-income countries. Posing themselves holding sick children or with disadvantaged community members may carry a different meaning in humanitarian work and suggest that we disrespect the people we are trying to help.

For years, communicators in the field of global development have been working to fight stereotype-reinforcing images in charity ads through awareness campaigns and codes of ethics. But few specifically address social media or are geared toward young people. One such project is the "Barbie savior" Instagram parody account, a project of the Norwegian Students' and Academics' International Assistance Fund (SAIH), which fights stereotypes in aid and development (Gharib, 2017). The staged photos depict a Barbie doll traveling to a low-income country and doing photo-ops on the disaster sites and in hospitals (Figure 9.1). The "Barbie savior" meme quickly became very popular and many contributed to the Instagram collection of photos. According to the campaigners, the selfie-takers may not realize that their posts, from the photo to the caption to the hashtags, can perpetuate stereotypes and rob the subjects of dignity or privacy. As Beathe Ogard,

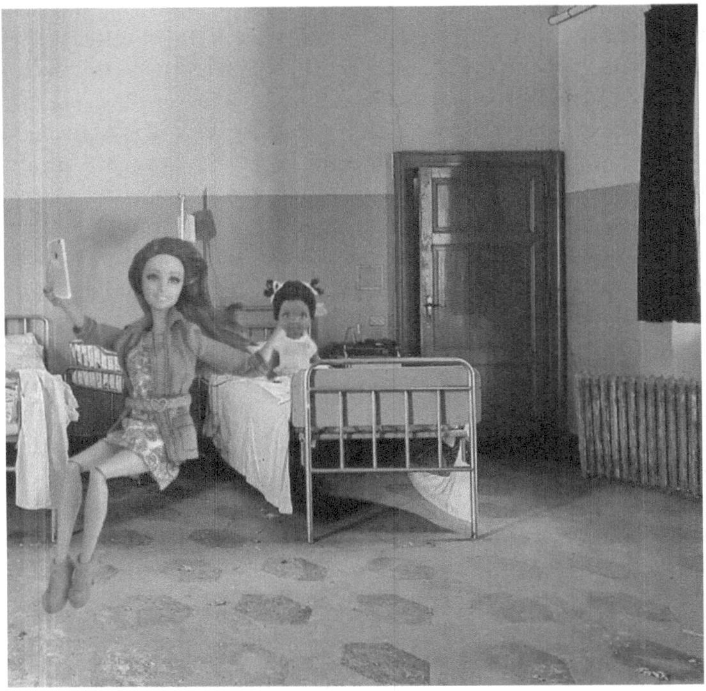

Figure 9.1 "Barbie Savior" (www.barbiesavior.com, used with permission)

president of SAIH in Norway says, a seemingly innocent selfie with African children, for example, can perpetuate the idea that only Western aid, charity, and intervention can "save the world." Ogard contends that these children are portrayed as helpless and pitiful, while the volunteer is made out to be the superhero who will rescue them from their misery (cited in Gharib, 2017). However there have also been concerns voiced by some who saw misogyny in these photos as depicting "a sexist and sexualized cartoon version of a female volunteer and used essentialist negative stereotypes to demonize her as an airheaded bimbo" (https://sm4good.com/2017/11/10/new-social-media-guide-for-volunteers-and-travellers).

To raise awareness of the sensitive issues around social media, the Norwegian Students' and Academics' International Assistance Fund (SAIH) has published a short guide that aims to make people pause—and maybe even ask for consent—before posting the next selfie with a group of poor children (see Figure 9.2).

"Disaster Tourism" or "Trauma Tourism"

Disaster or trauma tourism doesn't have a formal definition, yet its connotation refers to spectators who flock to places of disaster to voyeuristically watch destruction and suffering for thrill-seeking or other psychological gain.

This phenomenon was powerfully described by C. L. Moore in the 1946 science fiction novel *Vintage Season*, which revolves around voyeuristic rich time travelers who organize their entertainment tours to visit the most horrifying disaster scenes right before the disasters happen. The travelers must agree to certain contractual rules: they are not to develop any personal connections or intervene because this may change the sequence of historical events. They can, however, collect souvenirs, and they feel that touring the disasters helps them to cope with boredom, meaninglessness, and depression because they start appreciating their own lives more.

A newer side of trauma tourism includes providers who travel "to help sufferers" by bringing books on psychology or spiritualism, teaching them "how to dance or do crafts," use "evidence-based practices," or just "make them happy" by interviewing them and giving the opportunity to share their stories; or prescribers who drop by to prescribe psychotropic medications; or researchers who collect and publish data with little regard for the safety of the research subjects or sharing their data with the community.

While human curiosity is an understandable motivation to travel, those visiting impoverished or disaster-stricken regions must be attuned to the cost–benefit ratio. When planning a trip, I encourage providers to ask themselves whether this trip benefits the population in need in a greater way than would just donating the funds that they would have spent on travel.

"Playing God"

In the field, expatriate GMH providers possess tremendous power in making life-or-death decisions about the people they serve, and humanitarian agencies

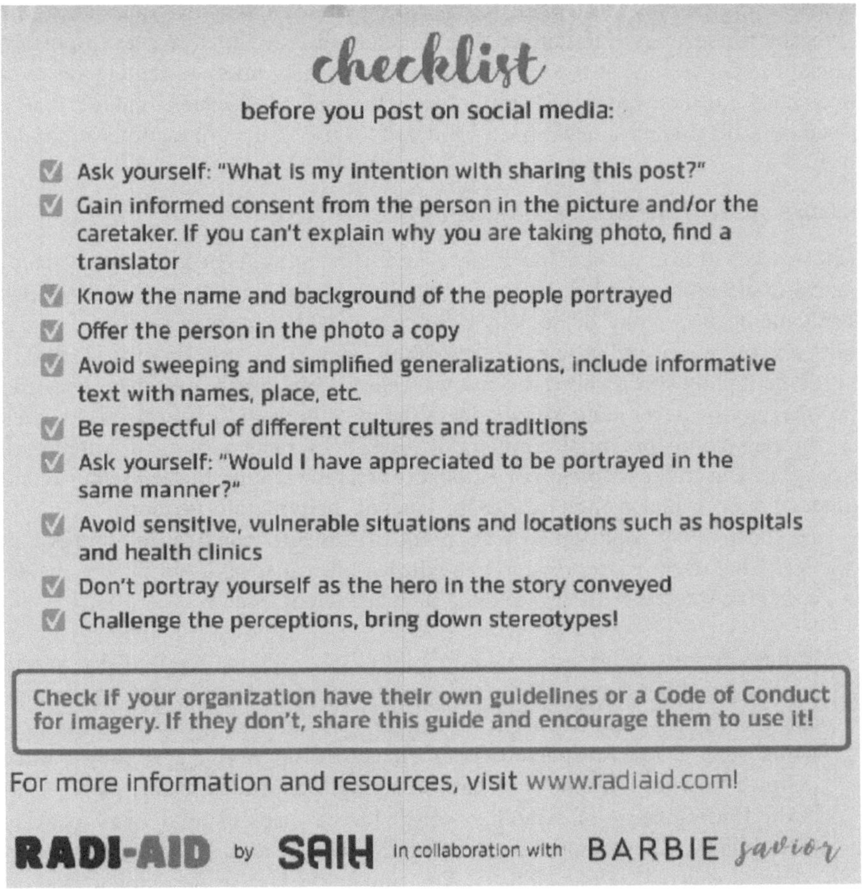

Figure 9.2 How to Communicate with the World: A Social Media Guide for Volunteers and Travelers (SAIH/Radi-Aid. www.rustyradiator.com/social-media-guide, used with permission)

take their opinions and recommendations very seriously. It is not uncommon for clinicians to be asked for their professional input for a variety of reasons—sometimes for care coordination, sometimes because they were the only ones who knew the clients and were willing to advocate for their needs in understandable terms. At the same time, in a GMH context, this good deed can misfire: what if the advocacy will be used to prioritize clients for an evacuation, or to determine eligibility for granting asylum? Can we really guarantee that we know these individuals well enough? The flipside of good intentions can also be that because of this advocacy, other people with more pressing needs may stay behind only because they were not served by this particular psychologist. For providers, this power to choose who deserves to be helped can create extremely sensitive dilemmas. The advocacy for severely traumatized and mentally ill individuals are an important part of the GMH role; at the same time, MH providers must be acutely aware of the ethical considerations and implications for real-life decision-making that is based on tools that have never been validated for use in the populations at hand.

Misuse of Medication: "Feel Better" Pill

Scholars who have studied the history and current state of psychopharmacological treatments in global psychiatry have raised concerns that our knowledge about medications may be socially constructed and extremely receptive to the influence of money and power (Cohen, 2009; Safer, 2002; Schulman et al., 2002). Fundamental questions about the cultural relevance of psychiatric diagnoses and the integrity of developing knowledge about psychotropic medications, as well as concerns about potential conflicts of interest by pharmaceutical companies, expectedly add to the suspicion of a global conspiracy around hidden political and financial neocolonial agendas under the label of "helping interventions."

This controversy is particularly apparent in strategies for treating depression. The WHO has declared depression to be the leading cause of disability worldwide, and a major contributor to the overall global burden of disease.

> Today, depression is estimated to affect 350 million people. The World Mental Health Survey conducted in 17 countries found that on average about 1 in 20 people reported having an episode of depression in the previous year. Depressive disorders often start at a young age; they reduce people's functioning and often are recurring. For these reasons, depression is the leading cause of disability worldwide in terms of total years lost due to disability. The demand for curbing depression and other mental health conditions is on the rise globally. A recent World Health Assembly called on the World Health Organization and its member states to take action in this direction.
>
> (WHO, 2012)

Marcus, Yasamy, van Ommeren, Chisholm, and Saxena (2012) reviewed different protocols in depression treatments in multicultural environments and concluded that antidepressants can be an effective form of treatment for moderate to severe depression but should not be the first line of treatment for cases of mild or subthreshold depression—multimodal culturally appropriate supports, problem solving, and addressing the underlying social and political stresses were shown to be more effective.

The proliferation of psychotropic medications in LLIMC without proper control and accompanied psychoeducation irreversibly changes the mindset of the populations we are trying to help, as I observed throughout my experience: instead of focusing on building on their own strength and relaying the culture-congruent strategies to cope with the arising challenges, some are patiently waiting for the next supplement of "feel good" pills to arrive to the region.

Other ethical concerns revolve around the discontinuation of psychotropic medications, which is not unlikely in the unstable and highly unpredictable context of GMH work that makes it difficult to ensure consistency of supply. In addition, difficulties in monitoring adherence to treatment along with the side effects, complicate making decisions about lesser harm: taking medications versus not taking them at all.

CHAPTER 10

Safety Imperative and Self-Care

10.1 Mental Health Impact of Humanitarian Work

It comes as no surprise that the demands of fieldwork, exposure to mass suffering, moral ambiguities, and personal risks affect the psychological well-being and MH of aid workers.

According to Aid Worker Security Database (AWSD), in 2016, 158 major attacks against aid operations occurred, in which 101 aid workers were killed, 98 wounded, and 89 kidnapped (Stoddard, Harmer, & Czwarno, 2017, p. 2). In an effort to reduce violence against humanitarians, the World Health Organization (WHO) has launched a real-life interactive database to reveal the extent of violence against health care workers and the risks they face in some of the world's toughest places to deliver aid (Lieberman, 2017). The database, built in coordination with the International Federation of Red Cross (IFRC) and Médecins Sans Frontières (MSF), among other partners, was designed to collect and post reports of attacks from multiple sources as they roll in. Kenney, the acting chief of staff for the WHO's emergency director, who is overseeing construction of the database, told Devex (the media platform for the global development community) in a phone interview:

> When we can start to get the information out there, it can be used to understand the extent and nature of the problem, related trends, then we can advocate for change and target our humanitarian interventions to reduce the likelihoods of attacks.
>
> (Lieberman, 2017)

The standards that international law adopted at the Geneva Convention in 1949 state that civilians have to be protected in armed conflicts and war. However, despite their neutrality, aid workers increasingly find themselves caught up in political, ethnic, and religious tensions, are subjected to the growing risks and become targets themselves (Omidian & Panter-Brick, 2015).

An article published in the *Express Tribune* (2013) gives a poignant account of the aid workers in Pakistan whose safety is severely compromised by politics.

After the gunmen killed seven aid workers with local NGO Support With Working Solution (SWWS) in the Swabi District on January 1, 2013, Chris Cork, country security adviser for the UK-based NGO Abaseen Foundation, said, "security threats are at an all-time high. I have never in almost 20 years known things as bad as this." The author traces the origins of the spike in hostility to the militants' fear that NGO or health workers could be spies and that they may be spreading into other realms, an allegation that predates 2011, but that was reinforced by the death of former Al-Qaeda leader Osama Bin Laden in May of that year, and called for more state protection.

The data on prevalence of resultant MH issues among humanitarian workers varies significantly dependently on the methodology of studies and the assessment tools. Connorton, Perry, Hemenway, and Miller (2012, p. 142) examined 12 studies on relief workers and 5 studies on organizations that employ relief workers and found that the relief workers, compared with the general population, experience elevated trauma rates and suffer from more post-traumatic stress disorder, depression, and anxiety.

Furthermore, the Antares Foundation (Young, 2015) found that 30 percent of field workers reported symptoms of PTSD after field assignments and that 79 percent of the 754 respondents to the survey on the Guardian Global Development Professional Network stated that they had experienced MH issues. The overwhelming majority (93 percent) believed these to have been related to their work within the aid industry. In July of 2015, Brendan McDonald (2015), a UN aid worker, published an article in the *Guardian* where he described the MH crisis among aid workers and voiced the appeal to humanitarian agencies to stop failing their staff on MH and safety. On December 10, 2015, the United Nations General Assembly recognized the importance of this issue (United Nations, 2015), and McDonald initiated an online campaign to include issues around aid worker MH and safety at the World Humanitarian Summit, but this inclusion "has yet to be realized" (Maudling, 2016).

10.2 A Safety Imperative

Fieldwork does involve risks and can be dangerous. The NGO sector has recognized the growing concerns about the safety of aid workers and, according to Persaud (2014, p. 18), is currently in the midst of professionalizing safety and security protocols that call for common standards modules and accredited training programs for staff development. The importance of managing risks places the safety imperative at the center of these efforts.

In humanitarian work, the safety imperative or the absolute priority of safety refers to security and information technologies, environmental concerns, and the fundamental premise of how we assess the risks and prioritize safety. "Stay safe!" is what humanitarian workers often add to their goodbyes.

I used literature reviews, field reports, and the experiences of the attendees at my training workshops to identify the main factors that hinder compliance with the safety imperative (see Table 10.1). They are:

- the "dual loyalty" dilemma;
- the "humanitarian impunity bubble";
- "existential despair";
- a "rescuer fantasy";
- compromised personal supports; and
- burnout.

In helping professions, the safety imperative presents a particular challenge because it speaks to the core meaning of the profession, which is grounded in the desire to help others in need. This can be a reason why the "dual loyalty" dilemma—having to choose between ensuring their own safety and the duty to others—has always been an emotionally difficult choice for a humanitarian worker.

> For a provider–expatriate, following this rule in cases of evacuation, for instance, could mean abandoning clients and the work, and leaving behind co-workers and friends, which conflicts with the most deeply seeded professional, humanistic, and moral convictions. This can be extremely discouraging and traumatizing for aid workers.
>
> (E. Cherepanov, personal communication, March 16, 2010)

To address this contentious issue, the NGOs set protocols in case of emergency. For example, in case of a security breach, aid workers are expected to prioritize their own safety and the ultimate decision is made by the agency's headquarters (Bickley, 2010, p. 182; Sphere, 2014). Not surprisingly, this causes frustration, which is often expressed as anger misdirected at the agency, like blaming the agency for overreacting.

Based on that, I strongly believe that when it is too easy to lose perspective and feel that joining the victims is the only moral choice left, MH and peer supports, and the routine incorporation of the self-care and burnout prevention modules in the pre-deployment training can strengthen compliance with the safety imperative. Inclusion of the safety imperative as a requirement in the NGO code of conduct will contribute to improving safety.

Allan (2015) defines the "humanitarian impunity bubble," another factor affecting the perception of safety, as a false sense of safety when the rules and norms create reassuring and sometimes empowering perceptions of the apparently coherent and predictable spaces. According to Allan, the humanitarians live in their bubbles where they rely on rules and norms that are abstract and detached from the real-life challenges in the field—from laws or principles, to religious and biomedical values, to best practice and ethical guidelines.

Table 10.1 Factors Undermining the Safety Imperative

Dual loyalty dilemma	Having to choose between ensuring one's own safety and the duty to others
Humanitarian impunity bubble	A false sense of safety when the rules and norms create reassuring and sometimes empowering perceptions of the apparently coherent and predictable spaces (Allan, 2015)
Existential despair	A sense of the diminished value of one's own life as a result of witnessing mass suffering of existential proportions
Rescuer fantasy	A fantasy that the aid worker is charged with rescuing others, and that self-sacrifice is a small price to pay
Compromised personal supports	Conflicting or toxic personal relationship that leads to a feeling that no one waits for the aid worker to come home or cares about their safety
Burnout	A reaction to the overwhelming demands of the job accompanied by fatigue, depression, problems with sleep, emotional exhaustion, and taking excessive risks

I use the term "existential despair" to describe a sense of the lessened value of life as a result of witnessing mass suffering of existential proportions. The impact of "existential despair" on safety and self-care as well as burnout prevention will be examined next.

10.3 "We Must Not Multiply Victims"

"My life is worth as much as the lives of the people we help, and if they die, I die too." These poignant words belong to an aid worker who felt strongly that the true humanitarian commitment means equating lives of those who help and those being helped (E. Cherepanov, personal communication, November 18, 2013). Although this sentiment sounds high-minded and is consistent with basic humanitarian values and moral norms, it raises a red flag signaling possible confusion about the safety imperative. Not using all opportunities to stay safe can also have serious repercussions for the project and jeopardize the delivery of aid. Otherwise, this phrase should be formulated as: "I will do whatever it takes to ensure my safety before saving other lives. We must not multiply victims!" The slight difference in formulations actually means a profound difference in attitude, and sometimes a difference between life or death.

Exposure to mass suffering and mortality can lead to the impression that life has no value or meaning. This existential experience carries very real and practical consequences for providers and their work. The duty to the people we serve, the sense of overwhelming loss due to identification with victims, and survivor guilt, can possibly explain the aberration in the attitude toward self-preservation, taking unnecessary risks, and neglecting self-care. If not addressed, this perception can increase risks for providers and have a serious impact on their work and personal and professional choices: when a provider doesn't value their own life, it is difficult to explain to others that their life has value or to empower them to fight for life, sometimes against all odds. In my workshops and training courses, 75 percent of the participants with the fieldwork experience (N = 64) reported experiencing a sense that "in the field it almost feels like my life is not as important."

Empirically, I found it helpful to use two sentiments that help with injecting the reality check for those who have a difficult time with the safety imperative. The first one I learned from the first responders, and I came across the second one when providing psychological support to relief workers.

1. "*We must not multiply victims.*" In fieldwork, with its prolonged exposure to severe trauma and extreme suffering, it is not uncommon for an aid worker to take extra risks or be willing to self-sacrifice if it would help others. The "not multiplying victims" sentiment appeals to the rational level of moral decision-making by reducing existential questions about the value of life to simple math. It allows for objective criteria for finding a best solution in a situation with no good solutions, where tremendous moral pressure can compromise judgment.
2. "*My life does not belong to me only.*" As demonstrated earlier, a field worker cannot always rely on their own perception in evaluating risks: "In the field it almost feels like my life is not as important" (the statement of a returned volunteer). A reminder about responsibility toward family and friends who on the one hand are proud of their loved ones but also trust that they will do everything they can to stay safe, helps to expand the tunnel vision to incorporate the relevance of the world beyond their work. Unfortunately, this strategy of finding an external reason for prioritizing their safety has limitations, and may misfire if the family or social supports are compromised or nonexistent—which exponentially increases aid workers' psychological vulnerabilities.

10.4 Recognizing Burnout

Burnout is an occupational hazard in GMH that is exacerbated by professional and personal isolation, emotional drain from empathizing, long hours of work with limited resources and supports, and ambiguous success. Exposure to mass human suffering and moral conundrums can be traumatizing and triggering compassion fatigue. The literature indicates that professional helpers can develop subclinical signs and symptoms of PTSD following their witness of traumatic stress in clients. To capture this phenomenon, Figley (1995), Pearlman & Saakvitne (1995), and Stamm (1995) introduced the term *secondary traumatic stress*. Its symptoms include:

- hyperarousal (heightened reactivity—startle, heart rate, pulse);
- intrusive symptoms;
- avoidance or emotional "numbing";

- anxiety; and
- depression.

Secondary trauma and burnout in helping professions have long been recognized as causing depression, cynicism, isolation, boredom, loss of compassion, discouragement, emotional exhaustion, substance abuse, and a reduction in one's sense of personal accomplishment (Figley, 1995; Pearlman & Saakvitne, 1995). Everall and Paulson (2004) outlined the impact of burnout on ethical behavior, noting that burnout and secondary traumatic stress diminish the ability to function professionally, which may place clients at risk and thus constitutes a serious violation of the ethical principles. The National Center for PTSD (s.v. "burnout") has noted that burnout often manifests as a gradual wearing down over time and that contributing factors include:

- professional isolation;
- emotional drain from empathizing;
- difficult client population;
- long hours with few resources;
- ambiguous success;
- unreciprocated giving and attentiveness;
- failure to live up to one's own expectations for effecting positive change.

Cherepanov (2017a) identified additional factors contributing to cases of occupational burnout in the fieldwork:

- physical hardship;
- lack of safety;
- lack of privacy;
- personal traumatization as a result of threats or attacks;
- exposure to extreme trauma, mass suffering, and mortality;
- complex moral and professional dilemmas and difficult moral choices;
- feeling that work is meaningless in the face of overwhelming needs;
- not being able to help everyone who needs help;
- limited resources;
- pre-deployment problems: social, MH, conflicts with friends or family;
- failure of mission when a provider is not able to complete the mission agenda.

Exposure to suffering of existential proportions is a reminder of the fragility of life and plants the fear that the work is not going to change anything and is done in vain. This realization can trigger existential crises including questions about the purpose of the work and the value of life.

In addition to the signs of burnout introduced in the sources mentioned above, Table 10.2 describes additional indicators of burnout as per field workers' reports, along with contributing factors (E. Cherepanov, personal

Table 10.2 Burnout: Indicators and Contributing Causes

Behavioral Indicators	*Contributing Experience*
Questioning the meaning of life and work	Existential despair and existential fatigue
Misanthropic attitude	
Loss of faith in humanity	
Social isolation	Depression
Loss of motivation to work	
Loss of meaning of work: "nothing will make a difference"	
Self-neglect, e.g. not being able to eat when others don't have enough food	Survivor guilt
Recklessness and excessive risk taking	
Feeling that your own life is not as important when so many other people die	
Excessive anger and criticism toward the deploying organization, which is misdirected and, in fact, should be addressed toward injustice and suffering. The organization may be imperfect, but it is there to help.	Helplessness, hopelessness
Identification with the victim or perpetrator	Countertransference
Victim blaming	
Rescuer fantasies	Sense of omnipotence and being irreplaceable
Increased stresses and conflicts at work and at home	Blurring the boundaries between personal life and work; between emergency and non-emergency mode
Family breakup	
Job loss	
Compromised support system	
Making life-changing decisions while in the field	Neglecting planning for reentry
Committing to the next assignment without taking enough time to recover	

communication, 2011–2016). These indicators do not reach the clinical level of symptoms, but they still significantly affect the quality of work and life, health and safety, and can result in depression and anxiety, maladaptive coping patterns, and psychological isolation.

Recognition of the impact of work-related stressors on health and wellness of humanitarians has already led to major changes. NGOs are now more than ever aware of the MH needs of aid workers and have been implementing psychological supports in various formats: predeparture psychoeducation, psychological support in the field (such as debriefings), and peer support networks to assist coping with trauma, stresses, and psychosocial issues during reentry. Large NGOs like MSF use crisis intervention services and external referral systems, such as employee assistance programs (EAP), which are made available to personnel to reduce the emotional burden of burnout and in cases of more extensive MH needs.

10.5 Burnout Prevention and Reversal

There is plentiful literature on managing workplace burnout: 143,000 results for the keyword "burnout prevention" were on Google as of October 1, 2017. At the same time, the vast majority of recommendations are hardly realistic for a field setting: some suggest spending more time doing pleasurable things, like taking a bath, lighting a fragrant candle, going to the gym or for a brisk walk, visiting friends, talking to loved ones, improving diet, etc. Figure 10.1 shows one such circulated poster that offers suggestions that could be helpful in regular life and work, but are irrelevant in the field. Similar posters are known to be read by humanitarian workers in their spare time as a form of comic relief, highlighting the incongruency of the recommendations to the nature of work.

On a more serious note, Everall and Paulson (2004) proposed three major avenues for burnout prevention: self-awareness, obtaining supervision, and peer support. However, many other things can be done as well. Table 10.3 includes a set of recommendations for preventing and reversing burnout, which has been developed based on field workers' reports and incorporated into pre-deployment training (Cherepanov, 2017a).

10.6 Reentry or "The Other Life"

Cherepanov (1999) described significant psychological challenges that returning field workers face during reentry, leading to lingering depression, interpersonal

1	Exercise—7 minutes may be enough
2	Sleep more—you will be less sensitive to negative emotions
3	Move closer to work—a short commute is worth more than a big house
4	Spend time with friends and family
5	Go outside—happiness is maximized at 13.9 degrees Celsius
6	Help others—100 hours a year is a magical number
7	Practice smiling—it can alleviate pain
8	Plan a trip—but don't take one
9	Meditate—re-wire your brain for happiness
10	Practice gratitude—increase both happiness and life satisfaction

Figure 10.1 10 Ways to Be Happier Today (10 Simple Things You Can Do Today That Will Make You Happier, Backed By Science. *Buffer Blog Newsletter*. https://blog.bufferapp.com/10-scientifically-proven-ways-to-make-yourself-happier)

Table 10.3 Strategies for Burnout Prevention and Reversal

1	Learn about burnout, its impact on MH, and the importance of self-care
2	Learn to recognize the signs of burnout
3	Create an inventory of your vulnerabilities, strengths, supports, and sources of resilience
4	Mobilize support and review coping skills that helped in the past, such as journaling, reading, arts, spirituality
5	Bring a non-professional book for personal reading
6	Use any opportunity to safely get privacy
7	Learn to accept moral ambiguity and things that one has no control over
8	Compartmentalize: as much as possible, try to establish clear boundaries between personal and professional life
9	Pay attention when peers express concerns about your psychological well-being
10	Do not make any life-changing decisions while in the field
11	Reach out and talk to peers, even if it's only about the weather
12	Discuss concerns about the quality of work life with the supervisor or manager
13	Plan for reentry
14	Take breaks between assignments
15	Reach out for professional help if symptoms persist or worsen

difficulties, social isolation, and even job loss, which further depletes much needed supports.

In order to adequately prepare and plan for reentry, a field worker needs to be aware of the associated challenges and know when and how to reach out for professional help. Many aid workers have shared with me that their reentry, or coming back home, was more psychologically difficult than going to the field. In the field, MH professionals cope with a wide range of stressful and traumatic experiences by compartmentalizing them or by emotionally disengaging from hardship and stresses in "emergency mode." The same compartmentalization can cause adjustment problems during day-to-day readjustment to routine life, when a person becomes emotionally numb and may not be able to fully engage in their personal life or job. Hodgkinson and Stewart's (1998) studies of emergency personnel confirmed that reentry can be psychologically challenging and associated with increased risks for substance abuse, depression, family breakup, or suicide. While stresses and trauma in aid workers now are being studied better (Young, 2015), the subclinical consequences of prolonged exposure to severe stressors still presents a comparatively new area.

In an earlier paper (Cherepanov, 1999), I examined the post-mission adjustment of returned field volunteers and described the following factors that by and large determine successful readjustment during reentry:

- good social supports;
- stress management skills and a sense of humor;

Table 10.4 Return from Mission: Normal Versus Complicated Reentry

Normal Reentry	*Complicated Reentry*
Attending to physical and mental needs: nutrition, exercise, meeting friends, taking time before starting work	Poor sleep, anxiety, depression, irritability that does not improve or worsens
Emotional responsiveness and interest in current events and social interactions	Social and psychological functioning is not improving or is getting worse
Ability to experience a wide range of emotions and pleasures	Increased social isolation and loneliness; socializing only with peers
Increased and enjoyable socialization	Relationships suffer
Thinking about the future	Difficulties holding a job, having low tolerance toward bureaucracy and perceived or real injustice
Field experience used for personal and professional growth	Poor sleep: trauma symptoms, such as intrusions, flashbacks, nightmares, and survival guilt, do not improve, or worsen
	Increased alcohol and drug use or smoking
	Sense that your place in the family and with friends was taken and you have no role
	Survivor guilt prevents you feeling happy: "How can I be happy when so many people suffer?"
	Getting angry at those who waste food
	Feeling "stuck in the past"—thinking and talking only about the mission
	Feeling that life is boring or meaningless
	Trying to get back to the mission right away

- physical health;
- adaptive coping strategies, e.g. talking to friends, exercising, expressive arts;
- problem-solving and conflict resolution skills;
- cognitive flexibility: ability to accept others' views and opinions;
- secure employment and housing;
- being able to use acquired skills for professional advancement.

That study demonstrated that there can be a "normal" but still difficult readjustment and a complicated readjustment that requires a higher level of professional help. Table 10.4 compares these two kinds of adjustment.

Hodgkinson and Stewart (1998), Orsillo, Roemer, Litz, Ehlich, and Friedman (1998), and Koppel (2002) have also demonstrated that a great majority of responders never ask for professional help and are certain that they would never use their own agencies for this. They proposed that the peer support network plays a crucial role in promoting positive adjustment and strengthening access to behavioral health for those who need more supports.

10.7 Exercises: Preparing for Reentry

This exercise consists of two parts, stress management and burnout reversal.

1. *Stress management*—individual work.

   Create an inventory of your strengths and supports. To do this, write the answers to the following questions:

   a. What are the symptoms that you are stressed out?
   b. How do you cope with stresses?
   c. What is your personal strength that has been helping to overcome difficult times (e.g. sense of humor, hope, feeling of responsibility towards family, love etc.)?
   d. What helps you to relax and what do you enjoy doing?

2. *Burnout*—small-group work.

   Divide into small groups. Write down the answers to the questions below. Discuss the answers with the small group and report to the large group.

   a. Have you ever experienced burnout? What were three signs? What did you find helpful at that time?
   b. Identify three people in your life who you can trust enough to share your feelings and experiences.
   c. If you could bring three small personal items with you to the field besides pictures, what would they be?
   d. If you could bring three books with you, what would they be?
   e. Imagine that your deployment is over and you are coming home. Name three things that you want to stay the same, and three things that you want to be different.
   f. What would be the first three things that you would do and who would you talk to first upon return?
   g. What are three signs that would indicate the need for professional help?

CHAPTER 11

Values-Based Ethical Framework and Core Competencies in Global Mental Health

11.1 Methodology of Ethical Framework

How Is the Values-Based Ethical Framework Organized?

The history of GMH and humanitarian action demonstrates that some values are changing to reflect professional developments, but the spirit of humanitarianism remains at the core of everything that we are doing. As previously discussed, the values-based framework is understood as a system of values governing practices in GMH. This system includes professional and multidisciplinary ideals, principles, and standards that are organized based on their primacy in decision-making. This approach allows setting priorities based on which decision produces the greatest good for the greatest number of persons.

This chapter addresses the dry but nonetheless important topic of how multidisciplinary and multilayered values are organized to create a cohesive, seamless, and complementary system that is both profession-specific and consistent with the ideals of humanitarianism. It outlines the methodology used in developing the ethical framework, establishes the role of values in decision-making and answers the following questions:

1. What are the characteristics of values comprising the framework?
2. How are these values organized?
3. Do these values carry the same significance in decision-making and if not, how are they negotiated when they conflict?

Principles for the Values-Based Framework

It has been proposed that in the values-based framework, different groups of values play different roles and have different primacy in decision-making: some are imperative (safety), others are binding (professional code of ethics), guiding (professional guidelines), or aspirational (humanitarian principles). For instance, the humanitarian values represent professional ideals, and the operational principles refer to professional standards; their misattribution, e.g. using the ideals as operational guidance, may do a disservice, similar to how the best intentions can result in greater harm if they are not accompanied by operational strategies based on professional competencies. Using a values-based framework, a GMH professional works toward minimizing harm and relies on best judgment and professional and personal competencies. Just as coordination between humanitarian actors has been recognized as the backbone of effective humanitarian interventions, the values guiding GMH work are also expected to be interconnected, consistent, and complementary.

- *Interconnected* means that the multidisciplinary and professional values create a cohesive system where the professional silos overlap, as oppose to fragmentation.
- *Consistent* means the values do not conflict or contradict each other. For example, professional values must be consistent with humanitarian values.
- *Complementary* means that together they present a comprehensive and flexible system that is relevant to different facets of GMH work.

Ground Assumptions

In order to provide ethical guidance for GMH, the values in the framework must:

- prioritize safety;
- be based on humanitarian ideals;
- incorporate accountability;
- set operational priorities;
- allow establishing of hierarchy or primacy of values in decision-making;
- remain true to both core professional values and the ideals of humanitarianism;
- avoid inspirational but overreaching slogans like "our goal is to make every person happy," "we must eliminate suffering," or "make the world a better place."

11.2 Values-Based Ethics: Strategies for Decision-Making

Harris (2013) noted that the decision-making process in complex emergencies and post-conflict settings is often complicated and multifaceted, and if professionals attempt to simplify this process, they will likely be surprised by the outcomes.

As shown, the normative approaches to ethical dilemmas have limitations in capturing the complexity of multidisciplinary and multifactorial problems in GMH. To the contrary, the proposed values-based approach allows for balancing faithfulness to professional values with flexibility, thinking outside of the box, and situational appropriateness in independent decision-making. The values-based approach that is being proposed here is not a prescription for choices but rather the system of values that the competent provider navigates to make decisions with the greatest situational relevance. When negotiating conflicts of equally significant values, the hierarchy of values for professional decision-making in the multidisciplinary humanitarian context is established based on:

- "seeing the bigger picture," or incorporating the interventions into the larger agenda to broaden the frame of reference, provide a different perspective, and see the contextual relevance in the decision-making;
- maintaining self-awareness to allow for reflection on how decisions are made and help to manage cognitive biases and preconceived notions;
- prioritizing choices that are consistent with the safety imperative and lead to lesser harm;
- preferring decisions that contribute to establishing collaborations, consistency of interventions, and accountability.

The values-based approach allows us to tailor strategies to different kinds of dilemmas depending on the nature of conflicting values, which can be multidisciplinary, professional, or moral:

1. The competing *multidisciplinary* agendas can be reconciled by placing the dilemma within the broader context of humanitarian work and engaging a meta level of humanitarian values where safety is always a priority.
2. The conflict of *professional* values can be navigated by establishing humanitarian accountability as a point of reference.
3. The *moral* conundrums can be reasoned by exerting awareness and making informed choice about the appropriate level at which the decision is made: emotional, moral, rational, or professional.

11.3 Professional Competencies of an Ethical Global Mental Health Specialist

The American Psychiatric Association (APA, n.d.) has argued that GMH training in the United States varies across institutions and can touch on various topics including developing cultural competencies, learning how to provide service delivery in limited resource settings, understanding epidemiology in cultural and geographic contexts, learning how to navigate health systems and policies, and finding ways to improve access to care and treatment.

The American Psychological Association (APA, 2008) spells out expectations for US psychologists working internationally by stating that any prospective caregiver to an international community should work through an established humanitarian organization operating in the country. Examples of such organizations are the International Federation of Red Cross and Red Crescent Societies, UNICEF, Save the Children, and other humanitarian organizations. It also offered recommendations for the role of psychologists in the international settings who do the following:

- *Offer to provide information, consultation, or training.* Psychologists with experience in disaster mental health and/or public health can offer to consult with recognized humanitarian organizations and/or offer to provide training to international colleagues. We recommend working through established organizations, such as the National Psychological Association, or regional multilateral organizations and non-governmental organizations (for example, the International Federation of Red Cross and Red Crescent Societies). Should an appeal for help from psychologists come through these organizations, it is much more likely to have been coordinated with the necessary agencies and incorporated into the relief infrastructure.
- *Develop collaborative research relationships with psychologists in the affected regions.* Collaborative research relationships may assist local MH professionals in studying the psychological aspects of these events, laying groundwork for an even more effective response to future events. The effective assessment of psychological needs and resources and the evaluation of interventions are areas of particular importance.

The APA (2008) further endorsed a list of minimum qualifications for prospective GMH providers proposed by the IASC (2007). According to the IASC, the well-intentioned MH professional (who is not affiliated with any organization) should be discouraged from traveling to foreign disaster-affected regions unless they meet the following criteria:

- They have previously worked in emergency settings.
- They have previously worked outside their own sociocultural setting.
- They have basic competence in some of the interventions covered in the guidelines.
- They have an understanding of either community psychology or public health principles.
- They have a written invitation from a nation or established international organization to work in the country.
- They are invited to work as part of an organization that is likely to maintain a sustained community presence in the emergency area.
- They do not focus their work on implementing interventions (e.g. clinical work) but rather "provide support to programs on a general level, including the transfer of skills to local staff, so that interventions and supports are implemented by local staff" (IASC, 2007, pp. 74–75).

What are the professional competencies that are needed to navigate ethical dilemmas in GMH? In their work, GMH professionals face situations with a high degree of moral ambiguity, with no historical precedence or existing point of relevance, and they have to rely on their best judgment and professional and personal competencies. In the absence of universal norms, professionalism means employing the post-conventional level of ethical decision-making, which exponentially elevates the role of professional judgment rooted in professional competencies.

Kohlberg (1976) described this ethical competency as the highest stage of moral development where the moral reasoning is based on abstract reasoning using universal ethical principles. Post-conventional individuals elevate their own moral evaluation of a situation over social conventions. In this way, the individual acts because it is right, and not because it avoids punishment. People who exhibit post-conventional morality view rules as useful but changeable mechanisms—ideally, rules can maintain the general social order and protect human rights, but rules are not absolute dictates that must be obeyed without question. In Kohlberg's model, the individual's own perspective may take precedence over society's view; individuals may disobey rules inconsistent with their own principles.

Responding to the call for professionalization in humanitarian assistance, Walker et al. (2010) expanded this list by including the universal competencies of multidisciplinary aid workers, which they broke down into *values*, *skills*, *behavior*, and *professional knowledge*. They recommended developing professional associations and suggested prioritizing the following areas:

> In terms of values, skills, and behavior, core competencies might include integrity (being ethically motivated and following the accepted principles of humanitarian action, including impartiality and independence), accountability (taking responsibility for one's actions, being accountable to and respectful of beneficiaries and their communities, being accountable for the resources one is entrusted with), empathy (demonstrating respect and concern for fellow workers, beneficiaries, and host countries), resilience (being adaptable), teamwork (being willing to learn and practice new skills to help get the job done), diversity (demonstrating awareness of cultural differences), communication (speaking, listening, and writing in a way that respects humanitarian principles and those in need of aid), and technological skill (seeking to master and use advances in technology that could improve the provision of aid). Core professional knowledge areas might include understanding the structure of the humanitarian sector, having a firm grasp of international humanitarian law and refugee law, understanding basic safety and security issues, and being aware of the mandates and principles of the key humanitarian organizations.
>
> (Walker et al., 2010, p. 2228)

Kohrt et al. (2016) approached the professional competencies through the lens of professional training in GMH. They identified five areas for values-driven training innovation: values, competencies, training experience, resources, and education skills

- Priority values included humility, ethical awareness of power differentials, collaborative action, and "deep accountability" when working in low-resource settings, regardless of the overall financial status of the country at large.
- Competencies included flexibility and tolerating ambiguity when working across diverse settings, the ability to systematically evaluate personal biases, historical and linguistic proficiency, and evaluation skills across a range of stakeholders.
- Training experiences included didactics, language training, self-awareness, and supervision in immersive activities related to professional or academic work.
- Resources included connections with diverse faculty such as social scientists and mentors in addition to medical practitioners, institutional commitment through protected time and funding, and sustainable collaborations with partners in low-resource settings.
- Finally, evaluation skills are those that build upon community-based participatory methods, 360-degree feedback from partners in low-resource settings, and observed structured clinical evaluations (OSCEs) with people of different cultural backgrounds.

Table 11.1 summarizes the professional competencies of an ethical GMH provider that have been proposed in the literature and suggested by the GMH providers in my workshops. These competencies are designed to be consistent with the values of GMH and can be used in a training or supervisory context. They are subdivided into knowledge, attitudes, self-awareness, and self-care, and are written to apply broadly to various work-related tasks.

Table 11.1 Professional Competencies of an Ethical Global Mental Health Specialist

Knowledge	*Attitudes*	*Self-Awareness and Self-Care*
Learns the regional history and geopolitics of the country they work in	Is able to tolerate moral ambiguities	Uses supervision and training to increase the awareness of personal biases, preconceived notions, and prejudices
Is engaged in continuous education	Is open-minded and curious about different ways of life	Is aware that the safety imperative carries priority over all other value and seeks supervision and peer support if this priority is being questioned
Has knowledge and understanding of humanitarian values and operational guidelines	Learns about cultures by how people cope with life adversities	
Is aware of the limitations of Western treatment approaches and the problematic cultural validity of some assessment tools	Is always respectful to beneficiaries, coworkers, interpreters, and the community	

Table 11.1 (Cont.)

Knowledge	*Attitudes*	*Self-Awareness and Self-Care*
Is aware that complex needs of affected populations call for complementary integrated and multidisciplinary interventions Understands advocacy for refugee needs and *temoignage* (testimony and bear witness) as important parts of GMH work Is aware that the community may not be able or willing to support some survivors, and that there is a need to link or engage supports outside of the community Is aware that in countries where it is not safe to trust people in power, the needs assessments and safety screenings are less reliable Is aware of various barriers preventing beneficiaries from accessing health care and services and makes efforts to address those barriers Is mindful that asking too many questions or insisting on trauma narratives may make clients feel unsafe and make them feel interrogated Is aware of the stigma of mental illness and makes efforts toward destigmatization	Avoids criticizing services the beneficiaries may depend on Seeks ongoing supervision and peer support	Is aware of the impact of traumatic exposure and physical and moral challenges on MH and the causes of burnout, and exercises self-care

CHAPTER 12

Ethical Considerations for Refugee Mental Health Providers in the United States

> In a world choked by violence, conflict, and disaster, more people are now displaced than at any time in recorded history.
>
> (Oxfam America, 2017)

Serving refugees helps MH professionals to gain global awareness and master essential skills should they decide to further their career in GMH.

The 1951 UN Refugee Convention adopted the following definition of "refugee" to apply to any person who

> owing to well-founded fear of being persecuted for reasons of race, religion, nationality, membership of a particular social group, or political opinion, is outside the country of his nationality and is unable or, owing to such fear, is unwilling to avail himself of the protection of that country; or who, not having a nationality and being outside the country of his former habitual residence as a result of such events, is unable or, owing to such fear, is unwilling to return to it.
>
> (UNHCR, 1967)

According to the Pew Research Center (2017) Fact Tank, about 3 million refugees have been resettled in the United States since Congress passed the Refugee Act of 1980. In 2016, the United States admitted 84,995 refugees. The highest number of refugees from any nation came from the Democratic Republic of Congo, which accounted for 16,370 refugees, followed by Syria (12,587), Burma (aka Myanmar, with 12,347), Iraq (9,880), and Somalia (9,020). Over the past decade, the largest numbers of refugees have come from Burma (159,692) and Iraq (135,643).

This chapter examines ethical challenges in RMH work and equips providers with strategies for navigating common professional dilemmas. Although some of the issues have been discussed previously, this chapter presents a complete, standalone module that can be used for training and supervision purposes. It uses case studies loosely based on real-life scenarios to examine the role of humanitarian and operational values in guiding ethical decision-making.

12.1 Refugee Mental Health: Current Developments and Professional Challenges

Current Developments

The influx of refugees resettled in the United States in recent years has increased global awareness of and interest in this population among mainstream MH providers, which has led to an growth in GMH programs and specializations in universities (the key words "global mental health, master program" in Google search turns over 600,000 references).

Studies of the impact of refugee resettlement on host communities have demonstrated that refugees enrich the social, cultural, and economic life in host communities (Taylor et al., 2016; UNHCR, 1997). The transition, however, is not always easy: in the process of integration, refugees must overcome cultural and language barriers, trauma, and depression, and cope with multiple losses and adjustment issues. Refugee mental health (RMH) services aim at improving the psychological well-being of refugees by addressing barriers to accessing health care and supporting their adjustment and integration. Today's RMH focuses on the development of evidence-based and culturally informed practices and incorporates paradigms of trauma-informed care, integrated care, psychosocial supports, and psychological recovery, summarized in Table 12.1.

MH work with resettles refugees who fled war, violence, and poverty carries many similarities with GMH work: in both cases, MH providers offer psychological supports to highly traumatized multicultural populations who have barriers to accessing services. There are, however, some differences. On the one hand, RMH providers are able to utilize established referral systems and available supports. On the other hand, this population presents challenges for a mainstream MH practitioner because of special and complex needs requiring "outside the box thinking," which is not an easy task in the heavily regulated and inflexible health care system.

Professional Challenges

Globally minded MH providers who chose to provide MH services to refugees are driven by the desire to assist the most vulnerable groups, support the humanitarian cause, and learn about the world. In their work, however, they encounter various professional and personal challenges and complex dilemmas. The severity of refugee trauma, their barriers to accessing resources, and the sensitive social and political realities of current migration trends force RMH providers to attend to dilemmas that are unusual for the routine clinical practice. Table 12.2 describes external, professional, and personal challenges in RMH work that I have identified in clinical work, supervision, and training.

Table 12.1 Current Developments in Refugee Mental Health

Paradigm	*Explanation of the Concept*	*Implications for Practice*
Trauma-informed care (SAMHSA, 2014)	SAMHSA's six key principles of a trauma-informed approach A trauma-informed approach reflects adherence to six key principles rather than a prescribed set of practices or procedures. These principles may be generalizable across multiple types of settings, although terminology and application may be setting- or sector-specific: • safety • trustworthiness and transparency • peer support • collaboration and mutuality • empowerment, voice, and choice • cultural, historical, and gender issues	According to SAMHSA's concept of a trauma-informed approach, a provider, program, organization, or system that is trauma-informed: • *realizes* the widespread impact of trauma and understands potential paths for recovery • *recognizes* the signs and symptoms of trauma in clients, families, staff, and others involved with the system • *responds* by fully integrating knowledge about trauma into policies, procedures, and practices • seeks to actively avoid *re-traumatization*
Integrated care (Gröne & Garcia-Barbero, 2002)	Primary care settings have become a gateway for many individuals with behavioral health and primary care needs. To address these needs, many primary care providers are integrating behavioral health care services into their settings. Integrated care may be seen as a response to the fragmented delivery of health and social services—an acknowledged problem in many health systems	Integrated care is a worldwide trend in health care reforms and new organizational arrangements focusing on more coordinated and integrated forms of care provision. The key features of collaborative care models are: • integration of MH professionals in primary care settings • close collaboration between MH and medical/nursing providers • focus on treating the whole person and whole family

Table 12.1 (Cont.)

Paradigm	*Explanation of the Concept*	*Implications for Practice*
Addressing barriers to accessing health and MH services: geographical access, availability, affordability, and acceptability (Jacobs, Bigdeli, Annear, & Van Damme, 2011; Cherepanov, 2016)	Various dimensions of cultural, logistic, language, and educational barriers to access to health care and social services impede health and wellness and complicate recovery	Development of complementary systems of psychosocial interventions, psychoeducation, and destigmatizing of MH problems
Community-based psychological recovery in complex emergency model (CBPR) (Cherepanov, 2016)	Strength-based approach carrying the idea that recovery to a large degree is determined by the quality of community supports	Partnering with the community Identification of community strengths and recovery resources Mobilizing community and mutual supports Education about needs of vulnerable groups

Table 12.2 Challenges in Mental Health Work with Refugees

External Challenges	*Professional Challenges*	*Personal Challenges*
Social and political context: anti-immigrant sentiments Funding Insufficient logistical resources: lack of interpreters, transportation, culturally competent providers Organizational influence: values, rules, regulations, and expectations from the providers	Working with severe trauma Multiculturalism Culturally different concepts of health and wellness Distrust of the providers Language barriers Complex needs of refugees: MH needs cannot be separated from social needs Questioning meaning and effectiveness of work	Countertransference Unique moral dilemmas Existential challenges: questions about meaning of life Survivor guilt

12.2 Values and Competencies of an Ethical Refugee Mental Health Provider

The values-based framework for GMH suggests that in their work, RMH professionals rely on professional codes and use the system of universal humanitarian values as a broader frame of reference. These humanitarian values do not replace professional codes but allow workers to maintain a global perspective on the issues that arise when servicing refugees. These values consist of the universal humanitarian ideals and operational guidance proposed by IASC (2007), which are summarized in Tables 12.3 and 12.4.

Placing the work into the broader context highlights the need for special professional competencies, which I have formulated using the providers' feedback in my training and supervision. An ethical RMH provider:

- learns about the history and geopolitical situation of the country the refugee came from;
- is aware of the limitations of Western treatment approaches and assessment tools in different cultures;
- is aware of the precedence of local laws over cultural traditions, and makes efforts to educate the refugees;
- is aware that integrated interventions allow us to address the complex needs of refugees more effectively than standalone services and actively engages multidisciplinary service providers;
- is aware of barriers preventing refugees from accessing services and makes efforts to address these barriers, like assisting refugees with translation;

Table 12.3 Aspirational Values in Refugee Mental Health

1. *Humanitarian imperative* means that all humankind shall be treated humanely and equally in all circumstances by saving lives and alleviating suffering while ensuring respect for the individual.
2. *Humanitarian accountability* has been defined as balancing the needs of stakeholders and a commitment to providing assistance, avoiding unnecessary and costly redundancies, and focusing on sustainable development and local capacity-building.
3. *Impartiality.* Provision of humanitarian assistance must be impartial and not based on nationality, race, religion, or political point of view. It must be based on need alone.
4. *Independence.* Humanitarian agencies must formulate and implement their own policies independent of government policies or actions.
5. *Neutrality.* Humanitarians must not take sides in a conflict, or engage at any time in controversies of a political, racial, religious, or ideological nature.
6. *Not exploiting vulnerabilities*:
   a) *Proselytism.* This principle states that the provision of aid must not exploit the vulnerability of victims, nor be used to further political or religious creeds.
   b) *Sexual exploitation.* This principle proclaims that sexual exploitation and abuse by humanitarian workers constitute acts of gross misconduct.

Table 12.4 Operational Guidelines in Refugee Mental Health (Based on the IASC *Guidelines for Mental Health and Psychosocial Support in Emergency Settings*, 2007)

1. *Human rights and equity*. MH providers should promote the human rights of all affected persons and protect individuals and groups who are at heightened risk of human rights violations. They should also promote equity and non-discrimination. That is, they should aim to maximize fairness in the availability and accessibility of MH and psychosocial supports among refugees, across gender, age groups, language groups, ethnic groups, and localities, according to identified needs.
2. *Participation*. Psychological recovery should maximize the participation of local communities. In most situations, significant numbers of people exhibit sufficient resilience to participate in recovery efforts. Many key MH and psychosocial supports come from affected communities themselves rather than from the professionals or outside agencies.
3. *Do no harm*. Helping people affected by trauma can also cause unintentional harm when the interventions are not supported by professional competencies
4. *Building on available resources and capacities*. A key principle—even in the early stages of an emergency—is building personal capacities and strength, supporting self-help, and strengthening the resources already present. Where possible, it is important to build the engagement with available services, both government-funded and civil society capacities. At each level of need, key tasks are to identify, mobilize, and strengthen the skills and capacities of individuals, families, and communities.
5. *Integrated support systems*. MH interventions and supports should be integrated as far as possible. The proliferation of standalone services, such as those treating only rape survivors or people with a specific diagnosis such as PTSD, can create a fragmented care system. Activities that are integrated into wider systems (e.g. existing community support mechanisms, case management, formal/non-formal school systems, primary health services, general MH services, social services, etc.) tend to reach more people and carry less stigma.
6. *Multilayered supports*. In emergencies, people are affected in different ways and require different kinds of support. A key to organizing MH and psychosocial support is to develop a layered system of complementary supports and case management that meets the needs of different refugee groups.

- is respectful of interpreters and community workers;
- avoids criticizing services that refugees may depend on;
- is mindful about the power differential and the disproportionate weight given to their every word;
- is aware that refugees often come from countries where it is not safe to trust people in power (such as police or officials) and pays special attention to developing a safety plan—the lack of trust and consequent possible reluctance to disclose victimization makes safety screening less reliable;
- is aware that educating refugees about accessing emergency services is an important part of any MH service;
- advocates and raises awareness of the refugees' needs;

- is aware that a community may not be able or willing to support some refugees, such as the survivors of gender-based violence (GBV), domestic violence, or LGBT persons—in these cases, there is a need to reach out for supports outside of the community;
- is aware of the stigma of mental illness and internalized self-stigmatization, and respects clients' decisions whether to disclose MH problems—shifting focus to less contentious issues like problems with sleep or stress management can help to engage refugees in MH services;
- is mindful that asking too many questions or insisting on trauma narratives may make refugees feel unsafe and remind them of an interrogation.

12.3 Cognitive Biases and Self-Care

In the course of professional interactions, both MH providers and refugees carry preconceived notions, unconscious stereotypes, and misconceptions that reflect power differentials, personal experiences, and cultural or societal attitudes that may alter social perceptions. Countertransference, bias, and privilege erode therapeutic alliances and lead to inappropriate self-disclosures, judgmental attitudes, moralization, and diffusion of boundaries. Unethical practices can re-traumatize refugees, cause confusion, diminish their perceptions of safety, and make them feel used or taken advantage of. Although these biases are universally relevant to most multicultural work settings, the extent to which they impact the providers is exponentially greater when servicing refugee populations due to the severity of refugee trauma, the power differential between refugees and providers, and internalized societal attitudes. Only after MH providers become fully aware of and address their biases and prejudices can they truly account for and address the clients' misperceptions and attitudes, such as distrust of authorities or overcompliance, which may be detrimental to the quality of professional interactions in the MH setting.

Power Disbalance

The inherent and profound disbalance of power between a MH provider and the refugees affects the quality of therapeutic communication. For instance, the culturally engraved respect to the "White rich male doctor" (which I use as a symbol for quintessential privileges), can limit refugees' disclosure or their questioning of the provider's recommendations. An ethical provider who is aware of the power differential and acts in a responsible manner:

- pays attention to establishing trust prior to screening for potential victimization;
- is cautious with any recommendation or suggestion due to the disproportionate weight given to their every word;
- puts extra effort into ensuring that consent for treatment or release of information is indeed informed and not given out of respect to the provider.

Countertransference

The severity of refugee trauma carries a high potential for triggering countertransference, which implicitly or explicitly affects the therapeutic alliance. A competent and ethical clinician works on developing skills for recognizing and managing countertransference—one of the biggest challenges in MH and trauma work. Countertransference can manifest in various forms, including excessively strong feelings that are incongruent with the context or "rescuer fantasies." When acting out the "rescuer fantasy," a provider treats refugees as helpless, incompetent, and dependent people who have no recourse and who need to be "rescued." While refugees need as many supports as they can get, the providers must remind themselves that these refugees have survived incomprehensible hardships, demonstrated tremendous resilience, and are motivated to play an active role in their adjustment.

With this understanding, countertransference can be exacerbated by the following causes:

1. *Provider's personal trauma.*
   Example: After hearing a refugee's trauma story, the provider may experience reoccurrence of trauma symptoms such as hypervigilance, intrusive memories, nightmares, fatigue, or depressed mood.
2. *Identification with victim.*
   Example: A provider perceives a refugee as scared, vulnerable, helpless, and incapacitated—as someone who needs their hand held and guidance in every step because he/she would have felt this way in the presence of trauma.
3. *Identification with the perpetrator.*
   Example: In some instances, clinicians find themselves feeling angry toward refugees for being "annoying," "entitled," "ungrateful," or for "taking advantage of the system and our tax money." Such reactions can unconsciously reflect the belief in "a just world" or that "bad things do not happen to good people," a basic assumption we tend to develop in order to cope with unpredictability in life. This anger can also be a reflection of the adoption of anti-refugee societal sentiments, common even among those who have devoted their lives to humanitarian causes.

Biases

Biases are prejudices or preconceived notions in favor of or against one person or group (Oxford Online Dictionary, s.v. "bias"). Not all biases are negative, and certain positive biases may be the very reasons why some MH providers choose to work with refugees. Either way, only true self-awareness can mitigate the impact of these biases: We, as human beings, cannot be totally bias-free, but we can be aware of and manage them. Below are some examples of biases common in refugee work. Some of these biases and privileges have been described in the literature (those without reference have been proposed by Cherepanov, 2017a).

"Dominant culture" bias is the subconscious acceptance of the dominant society's racist views, stereotypes, and biases concerning one ethnic group.

"Ethnocentric" bias is in a way similar to "dominant culture" bias and refers to the tendency to view the world through the lens of one's own culture (Brewer, 2005). That is, individuals tend to judge others' behaviors, customs, beliefs, and attitudes by their own cultural standards.

The "host country" bias is the expectation that "they (i.e. refugees or immigrants) must be grateful that we allowed them to come to our country." It reflects a belief that guests must be held to a higher standard than the host population and that they can be considered feeling entitled if they request benefits or express dissatisfaction with their lives.

"Expert" bias is grounded in a faulty presumption of clients' incompetence and often manifests in treating them as if they were children. It reflects the underlying belief that the expert's knowledge and expertise warrants making decisions for the clients without discussing them ("They would not understand anyway" or "I know better what's best for them").

Privileges

Privileges are rooted in the power differential, which is an objective attribute of any helping setting because, by definition, helpers possess more power than those being helped. The Oxford Online Dictionary (s.v. "privilege") defines privilege as a special right, advantage, or immunity granted or available only to a particular person or group. This perception can be shared by both clients and providers. If not addressed, privileges can set the stage for abuse of power. Below are examples of common privileges. Some of them have been described in the literature and others have been referenced in the information space or introduced by the author (Cherepanov, 2017a).

According to McIntosh (1990, p. 5), "White privilege" is when Whites in Western societies enjoy advantages that non-Whites do not experience, as "an invisible package of unearned assets." This includes cultural affirmations of one's own worth and importance based primarily on race. The concept of White privilege also implies the right to assume the universality of one's own experiences, marking others as different or exceptional while perceiving oneself as normal.

McIntosh (1990) also defined "gender privileges," in relation to how for many who come from traditional cultures, being male confers an undue advantage to a provider who then enjoys greater respect from clients and is perceived as being more trustworthy.

"Information privilege" is expressed when a service provider holds access to information and has insider knowledge about the resources and the system. This provider is perceived as having the power to choose and what kind of information to release to whom.

"Socioeconomic privilege" refers to the perception that a provider is rich and has power due to higher socioeconomic status.

"Professional privilege" is the perception that doctors and other professionals have the power to make decisions for their clients by virtue of their role, position, and expertise and their recommendations must not be questioned.

Self-Care

A competent RMH provider, like any other MH professional, exercises self-care and uses supervision and training to establish healthy boundaries and increase awareness of personal biases, preconceived notions, and prejudices. This means:

- avoiding emotional over-involvement by addressing countertransference;
- balancing self-care needs with expectations for work and needs of clients;
- establishing healthy boundaries between professional and personal life and learning how to compartmentalize feelings at work, which includes avoiding using family members for venting and taking time before coming home from work after emotionally charged day (go for a walk, listen to music, take a longer route); and
- seeking supervision and peer support.

12.4 Case Studies: Negotiating Ethical Dilemmas

The following case studies provide examples of generic ethical problems arising in GMH:

1. taking sides;
2. imposing moral judgments;
3. making political statements or "importing civil war";
4. "playing detective";
5. cultural traditions or religious beliefs conflicting with human rights or local laws;
6. "I know what's best for you";
7. absolutizing self-care;
8. misrepresentation (e.g. speaking on behalf of a community or nation) or giving false assurances.

The hypothetical vignettes are loosely based on real cases. The goal of these case studies is to demonstrate how self-awareness and a humanitarian values framework can provide guidance in navigating conflicts of values and complex dilemmas. The discussion after each case offers practical considerations for the decision-making. The vignettes and discussion can be used for training and supervisory purposes.

Instructions

1. Review the vignette.
2. Examine possible reasons why the provider acted as described.

3. Identify the underlying conflict of values.
4. Make suggestions about how this situation could have been handled differently if "referring out" is not an option.

Case Studies 1. Taking Sides

A provider who works with refugees who have fled an ethnic conflict refuses to work with refugees coming from the opposing side of the conflict.

Discussion

Preferential treatment and siding with one group involved in a conflict can be an indicator of countertransference and can inadvertently contribute to community polarization. In addition, this decision is in disagreement with the principles of impartiality. According to the International Federation of Red Cross (IRFC, 1965), impartiality means that services and assistance shall be provided based on need alone and that providers must not discriminate on the basis of people belonging to a particular category, such as nationality, race, religious belief, class, or political opinion. It is recommended that this provider seek supervision or peer support to maintain the professional role and work on addressing barriers to the non-discriminant compassion toward suffering regardless of the refugees' role in the conflict.

2. Imposing Moral Judgments

After learning that the client used to be a child soldier who was involved in committing atrocities, a therapist requests a transfer claiming that he was trained to work with trauma victims, not the amoral perpetrators.

Discussion

Support for feelings does not mean endorsement of the behavior. The refugees we serve come from different backgrounds and have different histories. Some flee armed conflicts where they could have been involved not only as victims but also as perpetrators and may have done things they now are not proud of. People sometimes commit horrible deeds in order to survive or save their families. Moral judgment is hardly applicable to "survival mode," because we weren't there and we don't know what it was like or what we would have done ourselves to survive; hence, we are not in any position to judge. Perpetrators may be traumatized and in need of psychological recovery and rehabilitation. Exercising our professional role is extremely important in breaking cycles of violence. In such cases, an impartial MH provider with additional training and professional support can become a very important actor in assisting clients with social and psychological rehabilitation.

3. Making Political Statements or "Importing Civil War"

A clinician—a former refugee—places a political poster in the office that condemns the atrocities committed by one side during the historical conflict in her homeland.

A co-worker who is also a former refugee from the same region but who fled the conflict later has a different political point of view and feels intimidated.

Discussion

As a former refugee, the provider felt compelled to express support for the social justice cause and was hoping that this would increase trust from some clients. The provider's choice to express her political view, however, disagrees with the humanitarian principle of neutrality, defined by the International Federation of the Red Cross (IFRC, 1965) as abstaining at all times from participation in *controversies of a political, racial, religious, or ideological nature*. The principle of neutrality discourages service providers from taking sides in hostilities because the expression of any political views at work can be perceived as political propaganda. Although adherence to this principle is not always an easy task, especially when a MH provider also comes from a region deeply divided by civil or ethnic war, disclosure of personal political views impact clients and can also inadvertently instigate negative dynamics among the staff and the community where community attitudes frequently reflect the cultural beliefs and divisions in the country of origin. I have observed how communities of refugees, and unfortunately also the service providers, have been divided along conflict lines, and how a provider's endorsement of one side can increase divisiveness and the potential for reproducing the conflict on different soil, or "importing civil war."

4. *"Playing Detective"*

A refugee client provides an account of his/her experience that contradicts facts shared by other refugees from the same region.

Discussion

Edwards-Levy (2017) noted that Americans have a very long history of skepticism toward refugees. The current political climate has contributed even further to suspiciousness toward anyone who is different and has made it easy to lose perspective and succumb to the investigatory mode. At the same time, being truthful about the past is not a qualifying requirement for a psychotherapy client, and refugees have good reasons to be cautious with their disclosures. When unsure, clinicians should ask themselves how they would treat the situation if any other non-refugee client provided such conflicting information. Under the circumstances, unless risk assessment raises very specific red flags, the situation should be treated as a routine clinical encounter and not as an interrogation. In general, the immigration process is not conducive to health-related self-disclosures, and serious mental illness may be a barrier to being accepted in the country. For example, refugees from Somalia informed me that, in the 1980s, psychologists were employed to identify those who were disloyal to the government. In other instances, former military interpreters from Iraq and Afghanistan told me on more than one occasion that they were specifically warned that they were expected to take care of MH issues prior to being accepted as refugees (E. Cherepanov, personal communication, March 20, 2016). In treating refugees, the breach of confidentiality by the provider can be warranted only when there is reason to suggest that someone is in imminent danger. Nevertheless, the scope of mandated reporting must be discussed with the supervisor amid current safety and security concerns.

5. Cultural Traditions or Religious Beliefs Conflicting with Human Rights or Local Laws

a) A refugee client describes domestic violence in his family and explains that it is a cultural tradition, adding that his wife doesn't mind.
b) A refugee client whose child displays symptoms of serious MH issues declines referral to a psychiatrist and informs the provider that they will be using herbal remedies and traditional healers.

Discussion

Both of the above scenarios are examples of the dilemmas that arise when cultural traditions conflict with universal human rights or local laws. In such situations, the local laws have precedence, and cultural sensitivity and respect for cultural traditions cannot replace the requirement to be law-abiding citizens—mandated reporting must be exercised if there are any reasons to believe that a minor or a disabled person could be in harm's way. A MH provider who enjoys clients' trust can be instrumental in destigmatizing MH issues, helping their clients to reconcile traditional and contemporary values, and in educating clients about the law, which is an important part of a safe adjustment along with building skills in problem solving and conflict resolution.

6. "I Know What's Best For You"

A clinician suggests that a client leave her abusive and unemployed husband and offers support in placing her in a shelter.

Discussion

Giving life-changing advice in a professional setting is never a good idea. For one thing, this advice may carry a high degree of imperativeness for a client who also is a refugee, because the recommendation is given by an expert with many privileges (racial, socioeconomic, institutional, or host community). Privileges in the MH setting grant providers so much perceived power that clients may feel pressured to follow them, which changes the qualification of this communication from "questionable" to "clearly unethical." In response, a client can either follow the recommendation without questioning it, or (more likely) will put herself in more danger by limiting future disclosures. Awareness of privileges helps providers to communicate recommendations in a responsible and sensitive manner, which means that clients must be informed decision makers who are not treated as if they are children. The accountability principle underscores the importance of engaging beneficiaries in any decision-making about them: "nothing about us without us."

7. Prioritizing Self-Care Over Clients' Needs

A clinician feels overwhelmed by a client's trauma story and leaves the session to take care of his own emotional needs.

Discussion

Refugee trauma narratives can be emotionally overwhelming for providers who may feel that they need to take time out to regain control over their own feelings. Usually, in my workshops, about half of the participants believe that this is the reasonable thing to do. Unfortunately, unlike RMH providers, refugees are unable to escape their past and memories, and clinicians must be mindful of how their actions could affect the client and should therefore exercise contextual appropriateness, i.e. a "sense of stage." Sense of stage refers not only to what's being done, but also how the action appears in the context of a MH session. Balancing providers' and clients' needs helps to avoid re-traumatizing clients by making them feel unsafe or abandoned or confirming that their story is too terrible to share with others. Instead, the better option for a provider who is emotionally overwhelmed or triggered is to communicate this to the client and take a moment to cope with strong emotions without leaving the session and to resume the work after attending to their own emotional needs. Learning how to compartmentalize feelings is an important skill in trauma work, and following up with supervision and peer supports is strongly recommended.

8. Misrepresentation (e.g. Speaking on Behalf of a Community or Nation) or Giving False Assurances

A MH provider assures refugee clients that they are safe now, their ordeal is finally over, and they are welcomed by the host community or country.

Discussion

As much as we ourselves want to believe this, this information may not be accurate and can create a false sense of safety. While the refugees probably have left behind their biggest hardships and are likely much safer in their country of resettlement, they still must overcome many obstacles. The known phenomenon NIMBY ("not in my backyard!") is an acronym for a community that expresses compassion for refugees while they are far away, but becomes ambivalent when they land in their own neighborhood or town. There are known instances where a NIMBY attitude has triggered community tensions and hostility toward refugees. Instead, fostering realistic expectations, developing a safety plan, and providing education about how to use the local emergency services will better prepare refugees to handle unsafe situations. Subsequent use of supervision would allow MH providers to avoid emotional overidentification and wishful thinking that can blur professional boundaries.

CHAPTER 13

Conclusion and Future Directions

13.1 Summary

Ever since GMH has emerged as a professional specialization serving populations affected by humanitarian crises, it has been working toward developing effective practices and professional standards. Its accumulated experience has made evident that this work requires highly specialized professional and personal competencies, skills, and knowledge. GMH work in complex emergencies has challenged Western clinical approaches, highlighted limitations of normative ethics in global contexts, and underscored the need for a broader point of reference for ethical decisions where a GMH professional relies on humanitarian and operational values and professional competencies in ethical decision-making. The GMH increasing presence on the humanitarian stage has emphasized the pressing need for an ethical framework and regulations that would allow GMH providers to interface with multidisciplinary actors in a collaborative and consistent manner. It also exposed questionable practices such as ethnocentrism, pathologizing and medicalization of suffering, and disregard for the survivors' strength and resilience.

GMH providers often work in professional isolation in settings with complex and overwhelming needs. This work takes providers out of their comfort zones and exposes them to unique moral and professional dilemmas where they have to make decisions under duress. In these situations, ethical guidelines set up basic parameters for competent decisions about the best choice of intervention in complex situations. They strengthen professional confidence in making difficult decisions when there are no right or wrong solutions and help avoiding the ethically questionable practices. The high price for ethical violations in humanitarian contexts has underlined the paramount importance of professional accountability where ethics serve to ensure consistent and responsible care for vulnerable populations and the improved safety for providers.

The proposed values-based ethical frame of reference in GMH organizes multidisciplinary and professional values in a way that allows professionals to engage the broader frame of reference for the decision-making. The ethical framework for GMH gets its inspiration from the universal humanitarian principles reflecting the ideal of humanitarianism and the guidelines developed by the IASC (2007), which lay out operational directions for how these ideals can be implemented in practice. Providers rely on the system of values and the professional competencies in determining which situation-appropriate decision produces the greatest good for the greatest number of persons, families, or communities.

Global work exposes MH workers to unique situations that force them to reevaluate everything they thought they knew about the world and themselves. This experience has profound impacts, and can leave professionals questioning their professional competencies, moral beliefs, and the meaning and importance of their work. It comes as no surprise that this work greatly increases the potential for burnout, which affects the providers' health, puts them at risk, and diminishes their capacity to provide professional and quality care for the most vulnerable populations. This is a reason why so much emphasis is put on prioritizing safety, self-care, and burnout prevention, which are approached as ethical requirements. While NGOs are now paying more attention to the psychological needs of aid personnel and are putting support systems in place, there is a lot of work still ahead.

The analysis of history, the past and current challenges, and emerging themes in GMH have demonstrated the following:

1. The GMH paradigm is best defined by the humanitarian context, complex emergency settings, complex populational needs, and the modalities of interventions.
2. A brief but full history of controversies in GMH is reflective of a search for its professional identity, consistency, and standards of care in the age of humanitarian globalization. In its professional self-determination, GMH went through four identifiable phases: "good intentions" and fragmentation, integration that gave rise to integrated primary care and psychosocial models, diversification that demonstrated the need for standards and regulations, and a movement toward developing holistic and cross-sectional models.
3. With a scarcity of well-designed and culturally valid research studies and evidence-based practices, GMH specialists are now embracing the importance of developing a theoretical framework, standard of practice, and ethical guidelines.
4. Ethics carry critical significance in GMH, where professionals work with highly vulnerable populations in need, and unethical practices can put the populations they serve, as well as the aid providers themselves, at risk or jeopardize the provision of aid.
5. Ethical guidance ensures accountability, flags unethical practices, and assists MH professionals in negotiating complex dilemmas with no good solutions. When a person's worldview is shaken by exposure to mass suffering and severe trauma, ethics offer professional grounding and guidance.
6. Cherepanov (2017a) argued the need to broaden the frame of reference in global work because the professional code of ethics that serves to establish personal, organizational, and corporate standards and norms of behavior was developed to provide guidance in *most* situations. The values-based ethical

framework is better suited to guide professional decisions in *unprecedented* situations with a high degree of moral uncertainty.

7. The values-based ethical framework is a system of organized values, where some are aspirational and universal and some are operational and profession-specific. This framework allows us to establish consistency in interventions with other multidisciplinary humanitarian actors.
8. Humanitarian principles provide aspirational guidance and act as a living document that is evolving to reflect the conceptual developments in humanitarianism. Universal values are shared by the entire humanitarian community, where the main focus is on establishing humanitarian accountability.
9. The operations in GMH are guided by the guidelines issued by the IASC (2007), which provide operational guidance for a complementary system of MH and psychosocial support interventions in emergencies where the emphasis is placed on the development of multilayered and complementary systems of care.
10. Applying the values-based framework for navigation of complex moral dilemmas requires special professional and personal competencies to ensure that the interventions are implemented in a contextually relevant manner that is consistent with the core humanitarian and professional values.
11. Humanitarian research, trauma work, disaster response, community recovery, post-conflict settings, and fieldwork highlight different ethical challenges that require different strategies for managing them.
12. Reconciliation of multidisciplinary agendas in GMH can be done through engaging a higher level of values, where safety remains a priority. The accountability-based approach provides a point of reference in reconciling conflicting professional values. In the moral conundrums, self-awareness allows us to choose the most situation-appropriate level of decision-making, which can be emotional, moral, rational, or professional.
13. GMH work elevates concerns about the impact of any disbalance of power between providers from developed countries and LLMIC especially on the extent to which this can lead to substituting a true collaboration with a form of "missionary" or "civilizatory" help. Exposure to severe trauma and mass suffering in GMH makes providers susceptible to cognitive distortions such as countertransference, biases, and privileges, which compromise the integrity of MH interventions. Self-awareness plays a key role in managing this risk and must be addressed in the context of training and supervision.
14. The safety imperative means that the providers' safety must remain an undisputed priority at all times. At the same time, witnessing unimaginable suffering can lead to a disregard for one's own life and taking unnecessary risks. MH and peer support, and supervision, are important components in ensuring providers' safety.
15. In GMH, self-care and burnout prevention are not just professional competencies but also an ethical requirement. The professional and personal challenges

of GMH work put a heavy psychological burden on MH specialists, which, not surprisingly, takes a toll on their health and psychological well-being, challenges their ability as professionals to provide services, and complicates readjustment after the assignment is over.

13.2 Future Directions

The accumulated experience allowed us to reflect upon the achievements and shortfalls of GMH and to focus on the next steps, which include developing conceptualizations, evidence-based practices, and outcome measures.

Ng et al. (2009) believed that the Western models of MH that have been disproportionally skewed toward illness and disability and envisioned the future of GMH as a holistic approach arguing that all spheres of human life are interconnected and form a whole. In this model, the main goal of psychosocial interventions is viewed as inducing changes in all of these systems. Lately, there have been numerous publications reflecting the growing interest in this approach among professionals in the context of advancing the large-scale and cross-sectoral agenda, such as peace building (Bubenzer & Tankink, 2017; Rokhideh, 2017).

This book affirmed the central role of humanitarian accountability, the quality assurance and professional integrity, and demonstrated how the emerging professional ethics are tied to the development of the GMH paradigm. It highlighted and prioritized the needs-based areas for future development. These areas focus on the development of the following:

- Cross-sectional, holistic, and integrative approaches that would place GMH into a global context, such as recovery or peacekeeping frameworks, to help to overcome the fragmentation of GMH models caused by conflicting paradigms.
- Professional, community-wide, and multidisciplinary collaborations by achieving a common consensus on what accountability should be about in the humanitarian context.
- Strength-based recovery interventions that are culturally competent and attend to the complex nature of human resilience.
- Outcome measures to strengthen the accountability of interventions and supports.
- Best practices for GMH and standards of practice.
- Methodology that would synthesize the binary paradigmatic conflicts of values, such as approaches that would seamlessly integrate the response, capacity-building, and termination modes.
- A common humanitarian accountability framework that includes clarification on who GMH providers should be accountable to, as well as ways to implement and ensure the enforceability of remedial measures.
- Outcome measures, assessment tools, and research protocols that are ethical, valid, and culturally sensitive.

- Professional training on the ethics of GMH work, to include self-awareness and self-care modules.
- Guidelines for ethical psychopharmacological interventions in complex emergencies.
- Addressing the issue of discrimination within the humanitarian community and inequality between expatriates and national staff (salary differential, privileges, and career opportunities), which has recently become a center of debate. Addressing these issues has been identified as a prioritized direction in global action (Shevchenko & Fox, 2008).
- Improving safety, MH, and psychological supports for the aid workers. This is another prioritized direction for global action. These developments undoubtedly would require the concerted effort of the professional, humanitarian, and international community.
- It is recommended that NGOs strengthen the pre-, during, and post-deployment supports for MH and psychosocial service providers and include topics on ethics, decision-making in morally ambiguous situations, and burnout prevention and its reversal as part of routine training of GMH providers.

Patel (2014, p. 3) argues that the cross-cultural universality of international diagnostic frameworks for mental illness identified three major strategic objectives for GMH. They are resources, capacity building, and research:

> The first is to mobilize resources by advocating to policymakers, especially in middle-income countries that have more resources, to finance scaling up of mental healthcare [...]
>
> The second is to build capacity [...] There is a great need for investing both in programs that can build capacity that is scalable, and in curricula and other kinds of tools that can be utilized in these sorts of settings for these diverse professional groups.
>
> The third, of course, is research. We clearly need to continue to build evidence that focuses on addressing questions about how we can integrate evidence-based packages for care within routine healthcare systems, so that we can inform governments on how they can make their mental health programs more effective and efficient.

13.3 Conclusion

The global perspective on MH has expanded the horizon of MH practice and mainstream health care systems and reminded health care providers about their professional mission and ideals. Pearl (2017) identified three things that health care professionals in the United States can learn from global humanitarian NGOs to reconnect with the fundamental purpose of their profession:

1. *The power of mission* means *reviving and nurturing* a sense of purpose and camaraderie in health care providers; this would be a great place for our country to start.
2. *The essentials of organization*, which means learning from global organizations about a heavy reliance on efficiency, attention to detail, and cost-cutting, along with getting the right supports in the right place at the right time. If our nation did the same, we could raise clinical quality and make health coverage more affordable for all.
3. *The importance of clarity*, which means that there are no unimportant tasks if they improve health and wellness or save lives. During volunteer endeavors, all health care providers understand what they are doing and why: to save as many human lives as possible. It's hard to imagine a clearer "metric," and any step toward this goal is just as important.

In a short period of time, GMH, which started as a movement by idealistic professionals equipped with good intentions, has gained recognition as a vital part of international humanitarian relief. This progress largely became possible because of the professionalization of humanitarianism where adoption of shared values has established common ground for multidisciplinary actors to agree on basic principles and agendas. Placing accountability at the center of the cross-sectional governance of humanitarian response allows for the coordination of conflicting priorities and establishes GMH as an integrated humanitarian actor.

APPENDIX 1

Ethics for Global Mental Health: Training Curriculum 6–8 Hours

The training is designed for mental health professionals and those interested in global mental health and humanitarian work.

The content is planned for 6 full hours of instructions and exercises, which does not include breaks. With the breaks, it is suggested to allocate 8 hours.

The training provides knowledge of values governing the global mental health work, and equips providers with practical strategies for navigating professional dilemmas.

It uses self-studies, group discussion, and exercises.

Six modules are organized around ethical challenges that the providers face when providing mental health supports to populations impacted by the humanitarian crises, and emphasizes the importance of the safety imperative and burnout prevention.

Examples of the case studies for the exercises can be found in the corresponding chapters of the book.

Overview

When mental health specialists respond to global emergencies, they face unique ethical challenges and moral conundrums. Serving the most vulnerable populations calls for the highest standards of practice and places special demands on making independent, competent, and responsible decisions. In a situation with no good solutions, the humanitarian values and operational guidelines for psychosocial supports can provide a broader frame of reference.

The training is divided into six modules. It begins with the introduction, which allows participants to explore the idea of humanitarianism. Next, the review of the history and current trends in global mental health demonstrates how the quest for consistency and professional standards has emerged a priority in addressing professional and personal challenges. In the third part, after learning about the ground values of humanitarianism and the guidelines recommended by Inter Agency Standing Committee (IASC, 2007), the participants will practice applying these values in the complex decision-making. In the fourth part, the participants will learn about multidisciplinary, professional, and moral dilemmas, and practice different approaches to their reconciliation. The fifth part is dedicated to safety and burnout prevention. The training ends with a Q&A section, feedback, and suggestions for future.

Readings

Cherepanov, E. (2017). Ethics for global mental health specialists. Intervention. *Journal of Mental Health and Psychosocial Support in Conflict Affected Areas 15*, (1), 17–33.

Inter-Agency Standing Committee (IASC). (2005). *IASC guidelines for gender-based violence interventions in humanitarian settings.* Geneva: IASC.

International Red Cross and Red Crescent Movement (IFRC). (1965). *The fundamental principles of the International Red Cross and Red Crescent Movement.* Retrieved from: www.ifrc.org/en/publications-and-reports

Module 1: Introduction (30 minutes)

- Introduction of the participants
- Goals setting
- Training plan overview

Learning objectives. At the end of the sessions, participants will be able to:

- Learn about the professional background, level of expertise, and global experience of the trainer and the fellow participants
- Formulate the expectations about the training
- Gain insight into the humanitarian identity

Method: teamwork, facilitated discussion
Resources needed: training handouts
Visual aid: PowerPoint slide on the training objectives and plan
Activities:

Time	*Activity*
10	1. Instructor and group introduction, and expectation
15	2. The icebreaker
5	3. Training overview
10	4. Team work on defining of what it means to be a humanitarian
30	TOTAL

Examples of the activities:
Activity 2: The icebreaker

Objective: to facilitate the engagement in the training by allowing participants to learn about each other
Method: group work
Ask group to rank participants by

- the distance they had to travel to this training, or
- how much time they spent doing the fieldwork, or
- in how many countries they have worked

Activity 4: Understanding humanitarianism
Method: working in groups
Objective: to discuss the meaning of the humanitarian work
Instructions:

- Divide into groups
- Discuss what you value in humanitarian work
- Bring the results of the discussion back to the large group

Module 2: Defining Global Mental Health—Professional and Personal Challenges (60 minutes)

- Defining global mental health
- Historical periodization
- Current trends
- Professional and personal challenges

Learning objectives. At the end of the sessions, participants will be able to:

- Learn about global mental health as a professional specialization
- Familiarize themselves with its historical periodization
- Identify its external, professional, and personal challenges

Method: interactive lecture, facilitated discussion, working in groups
Visual aid: PowerPoint slides, handouts
Activities:

Time	*Activity*
10	1. Interactive lecture. Defining global mental health
10	2. Interactive lecture. Historical periodization. Current trends: professionalization and accountability
25	3. Group work. Identifying external, personal, and professional challenges in global mental health
15	4. Discussion, conclusion and summary
60	TOTAL

Module 3: Values of Global Mental Health Work (1 hour 50 minutes)

Learning objectives. At the end of the sessions, participants will be able to:

- Learn about the aspirational role of universal humanitarian principles
- Learn about operational guidance provided by the IASC guidelines for mental health and psychosocial supports
- Establish their interplay
- Practice decision-making using these values as frame of reference

Method: review of the materials, working in teams, facilitated discussion
Examples of the activities:
Activity 3
The exercise includes case studies from Chapter 6 (section 6.4)
Activity 6
The exercise includes case studies from Chapter 7 (section 7.3)
Resources needed: pre-training readings, handouts, PowerPoint slides, case studies
Visual aid: PowerPoint slides

Time	*Activity*
10	1. Review the humanitarian principles
10	2. Discussion
30	3. Group work. Using humanitarian principles as aspirational guidance practice decision-making in case scenarios
10	4. Review the IASC guidelines
10	5. Discussion
30	6. Group work. Designing interventions that are consistent with operational guidance
10	7. Conclusion
1 hour 50 minutes	TOTAL

Module 4: Navigating Dilemmas—Unethical Practices (1 hour 50 minutes)

Learning objectives. At the end of the sessions, participants will be able to:

- Recognize different kinds of dilemmas
- Use tailored strategies for reasoning in multi-disciplinary, professional dilemmas, and moral conundrums

Method: individual work, facilitated discussion
Resources needed: case examples
Visual aid: PowerPoint slides

Activities:

Time	*Activity*
10	1. Didactic training. Multi-disciplinary dilemmas
15	2. Individual practice
10	3. Didactic training. Professional dilemmas
15	4. Individual practice
10	5. Didactic training. Moral conundrums
10	6. Individual practice
20	7. Facilitated discussion. Managing ethical challenges in humanitarian research
20	8. Discussion. Unethical practices
1 hour 50 minutes	TOTAL

Module 5: Safety Imperative and Self-Care (25 minutes)

Learning objectives. At the end of the sessions, participants will be able to:

- Understand the importance of safety imperative and the self-care in global mental health
- Recognize the indicators for the burnout
- Know the strategies for its reversal and managing stresses of re-adjustment

Example of the activity:
Activity 2
The activity includes materials from Chapter 10 (section 10.7)
Method: individual study, team work, facilitated discussion
Resources needed: handouts
Visual aid: PowerPoint slides
Activities:

Time	*Activity*
10	1. Interactive discussion. Safety imperative Factors impeding assessment of risk
5	2. Individual study. Indicators of the burnout and contributing factors
10	3. Individual exercise. Burnout reversal and prevention
5	4. Discussion
30	TOTAL

Module 6: Wrapping Up (20 minutes)

- Conclusion: Q&A about the whole training
- Feedback
- Suggestions for the future

APPENDIX 2

Boston Globe Letter

A Sinking Sense of Familiarity As Another Aid Worker Falls

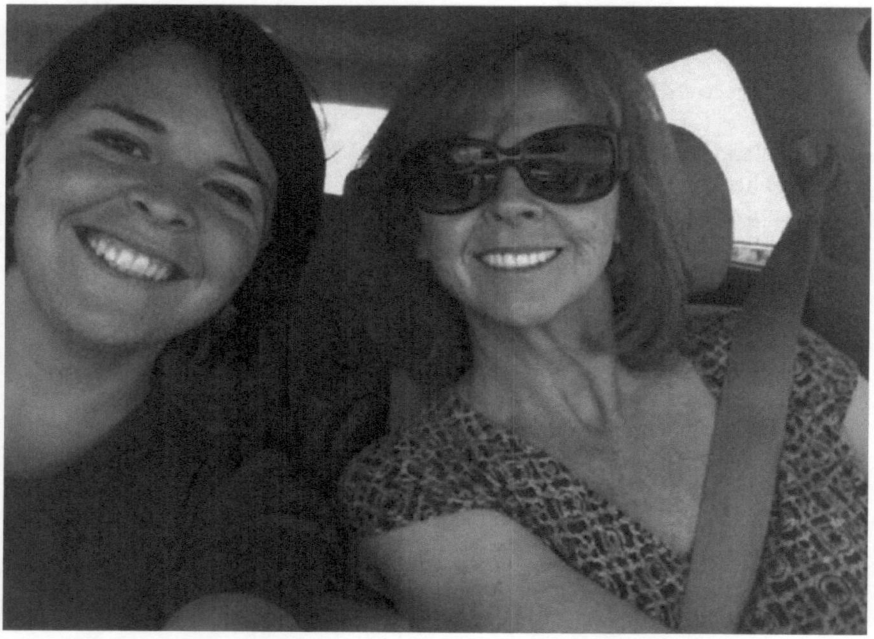

Kayla Mueller (shown with her mother, Marsha, in this undated photo) was taken hostage by Islamic State militants while working to aid Syrian refugees, February 10, 2015 (from www.bostonglobe.com/opinion/letters/2015/02/10/sinking-sense-familiarity-another-aid-worker-falls/UZWZw8tAdMDYqX4ygXKr7M/story.html)

As a professor who teaches about global relief work, I watched the news about Kayla Mueller, a 26-year-old aid worker, held by Islamic State militants, who has been killed, with a sinking sense of familiarity.

From Chernobyl to Liberia, I have known so many Kayla Muellers.

These young people somehow become relentlessly driven to find the very worst the world has to offer and try to make a difference.

I find myself asking why they choose this path. Even after being exposed to the real dangers of relief work, why do these young people continue, unfazed by the risks they know all too well?

I think of their families, dealing with watching their children go on missions, waiting and worrying, rejoicing at their return, and then driving them to the airport yet again. What is the future they see for their kids? Or has the horizon shrunk to simply the next e-mail or Skype session?

Every time I see a student's eyes light up at the description of my experiences, I ask myself if I am doing the right thing. What would I say to their parents if something happens to them?

I would have to say that the world needs them, we need them, and their families need them, too.

Elena Cherepanov
Boston

References

Abiew, F. K. (2012). Humanitarian action under fire: Reflections on the role of NGOs in conflict and post-conflict situations. *Journal of International Peacekeeping*, *19*(2), 203–216. http://dx.doi.org/10.1080/13533312.2012.665698

Abramowitz, S. (2015). What happens when MSF leaves? Humanitarian departure and medical sovereignty in postconflict Liberia. In S. Abramowitz, C. Panter-Brick, & P. Piot (Eds.), *Medical humanitarianism: Ethnographies of practice* (pp. 137–154). Philadelphia, PA: University of Pennsylvania Press.

Allan, T. (2015). Life beyond the bubbles: Cognitive dissonance and humanitarian impunity in Northern Uganda. In S. Abramowitz, C. Panter-Brick, & P. Piot, (Eds.), *Medical humanitarianism: Ethnographies of practice* (pp. 96–119). Philadelphia, PA: University of Pennsylvania Press.

Allden, K., Jones, L., Weissbecker, I., Wessells, M., Bolton, P., Betancourt, T. S., & Bhutta, Z. A. (2009). Mental health and psychosocial support in crisis and conflict: Report of the Mental Health Working Group. *Prehospital and Disaster Medicine*, *24*(S2), s217–s227. doi: http://dx.doi.org/10.1017/S1049023X00021622

American Counseling Association (ACA). (2014). *ACA code of ethics*. Alexandria, VA: ACA

American Medical Association, Southern Illinois University at Carbondale, & Southern Illinois University at Carbondale. (2006). *Code of medical ethics: Current opinions with annotations*. Chicago, IL: AMA Press.

American Psychiatric Association (APA). (1980). *Diagnostic and statistical manual of mental disorders* (3rd ed.). Washington, DC: APA.

American Psychological Association (APA). (2002). Ethical principles of psychologists and code of conduct (amended February 20, 2010). *American Psychologist*, *57*, 1060–1073.

American Psychological Association (APA). (2008). Statement on the role of psychologists in international emergencies. Retrieved from www.apa.org/international/resources/info/emergency-statement.aspx

American Psychiatric Association (APA). (n.d.) *Global mental health*. Retrieved from www.psychiatry.org/psychiatrists/international/global-mental-health

American Red Cross (ARC). (2017). Disaster mental health fundamentals: Part 2. *Participant guide. Disaster Mental Health Standards and Procedures*. Washington, DC: ARC.

Amstutz, M. R. (2013). *International ethics: Concepts, theories, and cases in global politics* (4th ed.). Lanham, MD: Rowman & Littlefield.

Anand, S., & Hanson, K. (1997). Disability adjusted life years: A critical perspective. *Journal of Health Economics, 16*, 685–702.

Arendt, H. (1983). *The life of the mind* (vols. 1 and 2). Boston, MA: Mariner Books. (Original work published in 1973)

Aung, K. T., 'Inayatibt, N., Rahman, A., Nurumal M. S., & Ahayalimudin, N. A. (2017). Ethical disaster or natural disaster? Importance of ethical issues in disaster management. *Journal of Nursing and Health Science, 6*(2), 90–93.

Balmer, C. (2017, July 12). Italy drafts contested code of conduct for NGO migrant boats. Reuters. Retrieved from www.reuters.com/article/us-europe-migrants-ngos/italy-drafts-contested-code-of-conduct-for-ngo-migrant-boats-idUSKBN19X2U1

Beauchamp, T. L., & Bowie, N. E. (1993). *Ethical theory and business*. Englewood Cliffs, NJ: Prentice Hall.

Behnke, S. (2005). On being an ethical psychologist. *Monitor on Psychology, 36*(7), 114.

Benatar, S. R., Lister, G., & Thacker, S. C. (2010). Values in global health governance. *Global Public Health, 5*(2), 143–153. doi: 10.1080/17441690903419009

Beyrer, C., & Kass, N. E. (2002). Human rights, politics, and reviews of research ethics. *Lancet, 360*(9328), 246–251. doi: http://dx.doi.org/10.1016/S0140-6736(02)09465-5

Bhutta, Z. (2004). Beyond informed consent. *Bulletin World Health Organization, 82*(10), 771–777.

Bickley, S. (2010). *Safety first revised: A safety and security handbook for aid workers*. International Save the Children Alliance. Retrieved form www.eisf.eu/resources/library/

Bobkoff, D. (2016). NGOs in Nairobi have to pay locals to attend meetings. MarketPlace.org. American Public Media. Retrieved from www.marketplace.org/2016/07/28/world/ngos-nairobi-have-pay-locals-attend-meetings

Bolton, P. (2001a). Cross-cultural validity and reliability testing of a standard psychiatric assessment instrument without a gold standard. *Journal of Nervous and Mental Disease, 189*(4), 238–242.

Bolton, P. (2001b). Local perceptions of the mental health effects of the Rwandan genocide. *Journal of Nervous and Mental Disease, 189*(4), 243–248.

Braak, J. (2002). *Ethics training*. Houston, TX: Annual Meeting of ATSS (training materials).

Brewer, M. B. (2005). Ethnocentrism and prejudice: A search for universals. In C. S. Crandall & M. Schaller (Eds.), *Social psychology of prejudice: Historical and contemporary issues* (pp. 79–93). Lawrence, KS: Lewinian Press.

Bubenzer, F., & Tankink, M. (2017). Introduction to special issue: Linking mental health and psychosocial support to peacebuilding in an integrated way. *Intervention 2017, 15*(3), 192–198.

Candilis, P. J., & Martinez, R. (2006). Commentary: The higher standards of aspirational ethics. *Journal of the American Academy of Psychiatry and the Law Online, 34*(2), 242–244.

Caplan, G., & Caplan, R. (2001). *Helping the helpers not to harm: Iatrogenic damage and community mental health* (1st ed.). Abingdon: Routledge.

Cavalier, R. (2014). Meta-ethics, normative ethics, and applied ethics. *Online guide to ethics and moral philosophy*. Retrieved from http://caae.phil.cmu.edu/Cavalier/80130/part2/II_preface.html

Charlton, J. I. (1998). *Nothing about us without us*. Berkeley, CA: University of California Press.

Cherepanov, E. (1999). Return from mission. *Trauma News*, *8*(4), 5–7.

Cherepanov, E. (2011). Psychological impact of radio-nuclear disasters. *StressPoints ISTSS online Publications*, *25*(6), 3–4.

Cherepanov, E. (2015a). It takes a village: Psychological recovery in complex emergencies. *International Journal of Psychology and Behavioural Sciences*, *5*(1), 16–25. doi: 10.5923/j.ijpbs.20150501.03

Cherepanov, E. (2015b). Psychodrama of the survivorship. *Journal of Psychodrama, Sociometry, and Group Psychotherapy*, *63*(1), 19–31.

Cherepanov, E. (2016). Role of the international trauma specialist in settings with complex trauma needs. In B. Ghafoori, Y. Caspi, & F. S. Smith (Eds.), *International perspectives on traumatic stress: Theory, access, and mental health services* (pp. 116–131). New York, NY: Nova.

Cherepanov, E. (2017a). Ethics for global mental health specialists. *Intervention: Journal of Mental Health and Psychosocial Support in Conflict Affected Areas*, *15*(1), 17–33.

Cherepanov, E. (2017b). Children as research subjects in global mental health. *StressPoints ISTSS online Publications*, *31*(6).

Chiumento, A., Khan, M. N., Rahman, A., & Frith, L. (2016). Managing ethical challenges to mental health research in post-conflict settings. *Developing World Bioethics*, *16*(10), 15–28.

Chomsky, N. (1999). Stop U.S. intervention: Noam Chomsky interviewed by Michael Lerner. Tikkun. Retrieved from https://chomsky.info/19990405/

Cohen, D. (2009). Needed: Critical thinking about psychiatric medications. In M. St-Onge & S. Dumont (Eds.), *Social work and global mental health* (pp. 42–56). New York, NY: Routledge.

Committee on the Future of Primary Care. (1996). Washington, DC: National Academies Press.

Clarinval, C., & Biller-Andorno, N. (2014). Challenging operations: An ethical framework to assist humanitarian aid workers in their decision-making processes. *PLOS Currents Disasters*. doi: 10.1371/currents.dis.96bec99f13800a8059bb5b5a82028bbf

Clark, J. (2014). Medicalization of global health 2: The medicalization of global mental health. *Global Health Action*, *7*(1). http://doi.org/10.3402/gha.v7.24000

Climate Change and African Political Stability (CCAPS). (n.d). Complex emergency. The Robert S. Strauss Center for International Security and Law. Retrieved from www.strausscenter.org/ccaps-research/about.html

Code of Conduct for the International Red Cross and Red Crescent Movement and Non-Governmental Organizations (NGOs) in Disaster Relief. (1994). Document. Publication Ref. 1067. Geneva: ICRC. Retrieved from www.icrc.org/eng/resources/documents/publication/p1067.htm

Cole, T. (2012, March 12) The White-Savior Industrial Complex. *Atlantic*. Retrieved from www.theatlantic.com/international/archive/2012/03/the-white-savior-industrial-complex/254843/

Collins, P. Y., Patel, V., Joestl, S. S., March, D., Insel, T. R., & Daar, A. S. (2011). Grand challenges in global mental health: A consortium of researchers, advocates and clinicians announces here research priorities for improving the lives of people with mental illness around the world, and calls for urgent action and investment. *Nature, 475*(7354), 27–30. http://doi.org/10.1038/475027a

Connorton, E., Perry, M. J., Hemenway, D., & Miller, M. (2012). Humanitarian relief workers and trauma-related mental illness. *Epidemiologic Reviews, 34*(1), 145–155. https://doi.org/10.1093/epirev/mxr026

Crittenden, C. (2016). Humanitarian innovation: Surprising news, cautionary tales, and promising directions. HuffPost Blog. Retrieved from www.huffingtonpost.com/camille-crittenden/humanitarian-innovation-s_b_9462358.html

Curry, D. R., Waldman, R. J., & Caplan, A. L. (2014). *An ethical framework for the development and review of health research proposals involving humanitarian contexts.* Report commissioned by the agency Enhancing Learning and Research for Humanitarian Assistance (ELRHA): R2HC Programme. Retrieved from www.elrha.org/wp-content/uploads/2015/01/FINAL-R2HC-Ethical-Framework_Final-Report_24-January-2014_0.pdf

Dagnino, N. (1996). Responding to the psychosocial needs of refugee children: A multi-faceted approach. In M. McCallin (Ed.), *Psychological well-being of refugee children: Research, practice and policy issues* (pp. 150–167). Geneva: International Catholic Child Bureau.

Darou, W. Kurtness, J., & Hum, A. (1993). An investigation of the impact of psychological research on a native population. *Professional Psychology: Research and Practice, 24,* 325–329.

DeGruy, F. III. (1996). Mental health care in the primary care setting. In M. S. Donaldson, K. D. Yordy, K. N. Lohr, & N. A. Vanselow (Eds.), *Primary care: America's health in a new era* (pp. 285–311). Washington, DC: National Academies Press.

De Jong, J., Komproe, T. V. M., Ivan, H., von Ommeren, M., El Masri, M., Araya, M., … Somasundarem, D. J. (2001). Lifetime events and posttraumatic stress disorder in 4 post-conflict settings. *Journal of the American Medical Association, 286*(5), 555–562. doi: 10.1001/jama.286.5.555

De Jong, K. (2005). Mental health overview. *Doctors Without Borders Newsletter.* Retrieved from www.doctorswithoutborders.org

De Jong, K. (2011). *Psychosocial and mental health interventions in areas of mass violence: A community-based approach. Guideline document* (2nd ed.). Amsterdam: Médecins Sans Frontières—Rozenberg. Retrieved from www.msf.org/sites/msf.org/files/msf_mentalhealthguidelines.pdf

De Jong, K., & Kleber, R. J. (2001). Early psychosocial interventions for war-affected populations. In R. Orner & U. Schnyder (Eds.), *Early interventions* (pp. 184–193). Oxford: Oxford University Press.

De Phillis, L. (2017, August 27). Red Cross volunteers deploying slowly, with conditions too dangerous to travel. *Houston Chronicle.* Retrieved from www.chron.com/news/houston-weather/hurricaneharvey/article/Too-dangerous-to-deploy-hundreds-of-Red-Cross-12034707.php

de Torrente, N. (2004). Humanitarian action under attack: Reflections on the Iraq War. *Harvard Human Rights Journal, 17*(1), 21–29.

de Torrente, N., & Stobbaerts, E. (2008). MSF and accountability: From global buzzwords to specific solutions. Humanitarian Practice Network. Retrieved from http://odihpn.org/magazine/msf-and-accountability-from-global-buzzwords-to-specific-solutions/

Dodds, P. (2017, April 12). More than 100 UN peacekeepers ran a child sex ring in Haiti. None were ever jailed. Associated Press Online. Retrieved from www.thestar.com/news/world/2017/04/12/un-peacekeepers-child-sex-ring-left-victims-but-no-arrests.html

Donini. A. (n.d.) *Sovereignty, globalization, and the future of humanitarian action*. Tufts University, Feinstein International Center (FIC). Retrieved from http://fic.tufts.edu/research-item/sovereignty-globalization-and-the-future-of-humanitarian/

Eaton, J., Kakuma, R., Wright, A., & Minas, H. (2014). A position statement on mental health in the post-2015 development agenda. *International Journal of Mental Health Systems*, *8*, 28. http://doi.org/10.1186/1752-4458-8-28

Edwards-Levy, A. (2017, January 27). Americans have a very long history of skepticism toward refugees. *Huffington Post*. Retrieved from www.huffingtonpost.com/entry/americans-refugee-polls_us_588b8ecae4b017637794129a

Ellis, C. (2007). Telling secrets, revealing lives: Relational ethics in research with intimate others. *Qualitative Inquiry*, *13*(1), 3–29.

Everall, R., & Paulson, B. (2004). Burnout and secondary traumatic stress: Impact on ethical behaviour. *Canadian Journal of Counselling*, *38*(1), 25–35.

Express Tribune. (2013, January 18). Helping hands at threat: Growing risks for aid workers. Post by PPI. Retrieved from https://tribune.com.pk/story/495505/helping-hands-at-threat-growing-risks-for-aid-workers/

Fellenz. M. (2017, August 30). Too little accountability creates monsters. Too much blame creates fools. *TheJournal.ie*. Retrieved from www.thejournal.ie/readme/opinion-too-little-accountability-creates-monsters-too-much-creates-fools-3570430-Aug2017/

Figley, C. R. (1995). Compassion fatigue: Toward a new understanding of the costs of caring. In B. H. Stamm (Ed.), *Secondary trauma stress: Self-care issues for clinicians, researchers and educators* (pp. 3–28). Lutherville, MD: Sidran Press.

Fischer, M. (2004). *Recovering from violent conflict: Regeneration and (re-) integration as elements of peacebuilding*. Berlin: Berghof Research Center for Constructive Conflict Management. Retrieved from www.berghof-handbook.net/uploads/download/fischer_handbook.pdf

Flannery, R. B., & Everly, G. S. (2000). Crisis intervention: A review. *International Journal of Emergency Mental Health*, *2*(2), 119–125.

Freud, A. (1946). *The ego and the mechanisms of defense*. New York, NY: International Universities Press. (Original work published 1936)

Geale, S. K. (2012). The ethics of disaster management, *Disaster Prevention and Management: An International Journal*, *21*(4), 445–462. https://doi.org/10.1108/09653561211256152

Geneva Convention (1949, 12 August|). *Document: International Humanitarian Law*. Geneva: International Committee of the Red Cross.

Gharib, M. (2017, November 26). Volunteering abroad? Read this before you post that selfie. Retrieved from www.npr.org/sections/goatsandsoda/2017/11/26/565694874/volunteering-abroad-read-this-before-you-post-that-selfie

Gillan, G., & Moszynski, P. (2002, February 26). Aid workers in food for child sex scandal. *Guardian*. Retrieved from www.theguardian.com/world/2002/feb/27/immigration.uk

Global Journal. (n.d.). Fresh look at the global governance. Geneva and New York. Retrieved from www.theglobaljournal.net

Glossary of Humanitarian Terms. (2008). Geneva: ReliefWeb Project. Retrieved from www.who.int/hac/about/definitions/en/ and www.who.int/hac/about/reliefweb-aug2008.pdf?ua=1

Goldberg, E. (2016, May 19). Doctors Without Borders ditches a humanitarian summit, no longer has "any hope." *Huffington Post*. Retrieved from www.huffingtonpost.com/entry/doctors-without-borders-has-lost-hope-in-summit-that-aims-to-reduce-human-suffering_us_5734d06fe4b077d4d6f26831

Goldenberg, M. J. (2005). Evidence-based ethics? On evidence-based practice and the "empirical turn" from normative bioethics. *BMC Medical Ethics, 6*(11).

Goodman, R., Speers, M. A., McLeroy, K., Fawcett, S., Kegler, M., Parker, E., ... Wallerstein, N. (1998). Identifying and defining the dimensions of community capacity to provide a basis for measurement. *Health Education & Behavior, 25*(3), 258–278.

Grand Challenges in Global Mental Health Initiative. (n.d.). *Document. Office for Research on Disparities and Global Mental Health (ORDGMH)*. Bethesda, MD: National Institute of Mental Health.

Green, B. L., Friedman, M. J., de Jong, J., Solomon, S. D., Keane, T. M., Fairbank, J. A., ... Frey Wouters, E. (2003). *Trauma interventions in war and peace: Prevention, practice, and policy*. New York, NY: Kluwer/Plenum.

Gröne, O., & Garcia-Barbero, M. (2002). *Trends in integrated care: Reflections on conceptual issues*. Copenhagen: World Health Organization. EUR/02/5037864

Hamre, J. J., & Sullivan, G. R. (2002). Toward postconflict reconstruction. *Washington Quarterly, 25*(4), 85–96.

Handicap International. (2016). Moving towards a major breakthrough for people with disabilities? *World Humanitarian Summit*. Retrieved from https://d3n8a8pro7vhmx.cloudfront.net/handicapinternational/pages/2224/attachments/original/1463689696/World_Humanitarian_Summit_PRESS_KIT_MAY_2016_EN.pdf?1463689696

Harris, C. E. Jr. (2013). Engineering ethics: From preventive ethics to aspirational ethics. In D. P. Michelfelder, D. E. G. Goldberg, & C. N. A. McCarthy (Eds.), *Philosophy and engineering: Reflections on practice, principles and process* (pp. 177–187). New York, NY: Springer.

Hinton, D. E., & Lewis-Fernandez, R. (2011). The cross-cultural validity of post-traumatic stress disorder: Implications for DSM-5. *Depression and Anxiety, 28*(9), 783–801.

Hilhorst, D. (2005). Dead letter or living document? Ten years of the code of conduct for disaster relief. *Disasters, 29*(4), 351–369. doi: 10.1111/j.0361-3666.2005.00297.x

Hodgkinson, P., & Stewart, M. (1998). *Coping with catastrophe*. London: Routledge.

Holtzman, S. (1999*). Rethinking "relief" and "development" in transitions from conflict: An occasional paper.* Washington, DC: Brookings Institution Project on Internal Displacement. Retrieved from www.brookings.edu/wpcontent/uploads/2016/06/1999_holtzman.pdf

Humanitarian Coalition. (n.d). What is a humanitarian emergency? *Humanitarian Coalition*. Retrieved from http://humanitariancoalition.ca/info-portal/factsheets/what-is-a-humanitarian-crisis

InterAction. (2012). Transition from relief to development. Retrieved from www.interaction.org/work/transition-relief-development

Inter-Agency Standing Committee (IASC). (2005). *IASC guidelines for gender-based violence interventions in humanitarian settings*. Geneva: IASC.

Inter-Agency Standing Committee (IASC). (2007). *Guidelines on mental health and psychosocial support in emergency settings*. Geneva: IASC.

Inter-Agency Standing Committee (IASC). (2014). *IASC recommendations for conducting ethical mental health and psychosocial research in emergency settings*. Retrieved from http://interagencystandingcommittee.org/node/9061

Inter-Agency Standing Committee (IASC). (2015). *Statement by the IASC principals on protection against sexual exploitation and abuse.* Geneva: IASC. Retrieved from https://interagencystandingcommittee.org/principals/documents-public/statement-iasc-principals-protection-against-sexual-exploitation-and

International Federation of the Red Cross (IFRC). (1965/1994). *The seven fundamental principles.* Retrieved from www.ifrc.org/en/publications-and-reports

International Federation of the Red Cross (IFRC). (1994). *The code of conduct for the International Red Cross and Red Crescent Movement and non-governmental organizations (NGOs) in disaster relief.* Retrieved from http://media.ifrc.org/ifrc/who-we-are/the-movement/code-of-conduct/

International Federation of the Red Cross (IFRC). (2014). *Performance and accountability.* Retrieved from www.ifrc.org/en/who-we-are/performance-and-accountability/

International Federation of the Red Cross (IFRC) and the Red Crescent Movement (IFRC). (1965). *The fundamental principles of the International Red Cross and Red Crescent Movement.* Retrieved from www.ifrc.org/en/publications-and-reports

International Humanitarian Accountability Partnership (HAP). (2010). *The 2010 HAP standard in accountability and quality management.* Geneva: HAP International.

Jacobs, B., Ir, P., Bigdeli, M., Annear, P. L., & Van Damme, W. (2011). Addressing access barriers to health services: An analytical framework for selecting appropriate interventions in low-income Asian countries. *Journal of Health Policy and Planning, 27*(4), 288–300. doi: 10.1093/heapol/czr038

Jayakumar, K. (2012). Humanitarian intervention: A legal analysis. http://dx.doi.org/10.2139/ssrn.2121008

Jenkins, R., Baingana, F., Ahmad, R., McDaid, D., & Atun R. (2011). Mental health and the global agenda: Core conceptual issues. *Mental Health in Family Medicine, 8*(2), 69–82.

Jenson, E. (Ed.). (1997). *Disaster management ethics, disaster management training programme* (1st ed.). Department of Humanitarian Affairs of the General Secretariat of the United Nations for the Disaster Management Training Programme (DMTP). Retrieved from http://reliefweb.int/sites/reliefweb.int/files/resources/2561747D821E0256C1256DB70053E6D4-undp-ethics-1997.pdf

Illich, I. (1974). *Medical nemesis: The expropriation of health.* London: Calder & Boyars.

Jordan, L., & van Tuijl, P. (2006). *NGO accountability: Politics, principles and innovations.* London: Earthscan.

Jordan, M. J. (2004, November 26). Sex charges haunt UN forces: In places like Congo and Kosovo, peacekeepers have been accused of abusing the people they're protecting. *Christian Science Monitor Online.* Retrieved from www.csmonitor.com/2004/1126/p06s02-wogi.html

Josephson Institute of Ethics. (2002). Making ethical decisions: A 7-step path. Retrieved from https://blink.ucsd.edu/finance/accountability/ethics/path.html

Jung, C. G. (1979) *Aion: Researches into the phenomenology of the self* (2nd ed.). Princeton, NJ: Princeton University Press.

Kaldor, M. (2007) *Human security: Reflections on globalization and intervention.* Cambridge: Polity Press.

Karadag, O. C., & Kerim Hakan, A. (2012). Ethical dilemmas in disaster medicine. *Iranian Red Crescent Medical Journal, 14*(10), 602–612.

Katz, C. L., & Schuetz-Mueller, J. (2015). *A guide to global mental health practice: Seeing the unseen.* New York, NY: Routledge.

Katz, P. A., & Segall, M. (1976). Towards the elimination of racism. *Journal of Social Issues, 32*(2), i. doi: 10.1111/j.1540-4560.1976.tb02490.x

Kidder, R. (1995/2005). *How good people make tough choices: Resolving the dilemmas of ethical living*. Portland, ME: University of Southern Maine, Institute for Global Ethics. Retrieved from https://usm.maine.edu/sites/default/files/core/How%20Good%20People%20Make%20Tough%20Choices-Kidder%20chapter1.pdf

Kirmayer, L. J., & Pedersen, D. (2014). Toward a new architecture for global mental health. *Transcultural Psychiatry*, *51*(6), 759–776. doi: 10.1177/1363461514557202

Kipling, R. (1899/1997). *The white man's burden*. New York, NY: Fordham University. Retrieved from https://sourcebooks.fordham.edu/halsall/mod/kipling.asp

Kodner, D. L., & Spreeuwenberg, C. (2002). Integrated care: Meaning, logic, applications, and implications—a discussion paper. *International Journal of Integrated Care*, *2*(14).

Kohlberg, L. (1976). Moral stages and moralization: The cognitive-developmental approach. In T. Lickona (Eds.), *Moral development and behavior: Theory, research and social issues*. New York, NY: Holt, Rinehart, and Winston.

Kohrt, B. A., Marienfeld, C. B., Panter-Brick, C., Tsai, A. C., & Wainberg, M. L. (2016). Global mental health: Five areas for value-driven training innovation. *Academic Psychiatry*, *40*(4), 650–658. doi: 10.1007/s40596-016-0504-4

Koplan J. P., Bond T. C., & Merson M. H. (2009). Towards a common definition of global health. *Lancet*, *373*, 1993–1995. [PubMed: 19493564]

Koppel, T. (2002). A good man in hell: General Roméo Dallaire and the Rwanda genocide. Interview with General Dallaire. *Speaker's series*. United States Holocausts Mem orial Museum. Retrieved from www.ushmm.org/confront-genocide/speakers-and-events/all-speakers-and-events/a-good-man-in-hell-general-romeo-dallaire-and-the-rwanda-genocide

Kreitman, B. (1996). *Bread, peace, liberty*. Lanham, MA: UPA.

Krell, R., & Eitinger, L. (1985). *Psychological and medical effects of concentration camps and related persecutions on survivors of the Holocaust*. Vancouver, BC: University of British Columbia Press.

Labott, S. M., Johnson, T. P., Fendrich, M., & Feeny, N. C. (2013). Emotional risks to respondents in survey research: Some empirical evidence. *Journal of Empirical Research on Human Research Ethics*, *8*(4), 53–66. http://doi.org/10.1525/jer.2013.8.4.53

Lambert, J. (2015). Ethical considerations for research with victims of political violence and human rights violations. *StressPoints*. Retrieved from www.istss.org/education-research/traumatic-stresspoints/2015-january/ethical-considerations-for-research-with-victims-o.aspx

Laplanche, J., & Pontalis, J. B. (1988). *Counter-transference: The language of psycho-analysis*. London: Karnac Books.

Larkey, P., & Devereux, E. A. (1999). Good budgetary decision processes. In H. G. Frederickson & J. M. Johnston (Eds.), *Public management reform and innovation: Research, theory, and application* (p. 170). Tuscaloosa, AL: University of Alabama Press.

Leach, M. M., Stevens, M. J., Lindsay, G., Ferrero, A., & Korkut, Y. (2012). *The Oxford handbook of international psychological ethics* (Oxford Library of Psychology). New York, NY: Oxford University Press.

Leaning, J. (2001). Ethics of research in refugee populations. *Lancet*, *357*(9266), 1432–1433. http://dx.doi.org/10.1016/S0140-6736(00)04572-4

Lerner, M. J., & Miller, D. T. (1978). Just world research and the attribution process: Looking back and ahead. *Psychological Bulletin*, *85*(5), 1030–1051.

Lewis, D. (2014). *Non-governmental organizations, management and development* (3rd ed.). London: Routledge.

Li, R. H., Wacholtz, M. C., Barnes, M., Boggs, L., Callery-D'Amico, S., Davis, A., ... Bierer, B. E. (2016). Incorporating ethical principles into clinical research protocols: A tool for protocol writers and ethics committees. *Journal of Medical Ethics*, *2016*(42), 229–234.

Lieberman, A. (2017). WHO readies to launch online database tracking health worker attacks. DeVex Online. Retrieved from www.devex.com/news/who-readies-to-launch-online-database-tracking-health-worker-attacks-90331

Lipsky, S. (1987). *Internalized racism*. Seattle, WA: Rational Island.

Lloyd, R. M., Blagescu, M., & de las Casa, L. (2005). *Pathways to accountability: The gap framework*. One World Trust. Retrieved from www.alnap.org/resource/8747

Locke. P. (2015) Anthropology and medical humanitarianism in the age of global health education. In S. Abramowitz, C. Panter-Brick, & P. Piot (Eds.), *Medical humanitarianism: Ethnographies of practice* (pp. 193–208). Philadelphia, PA: University of Pennsylvania Press.

Loewenberg, F. M., & Dolgoff, R. (1992). *Ethical decisions for social work practice* (4th ed.). Itasca, IL: Peacock.

Loff, B., & Black, J. (2000). The declaration of Helsinki and research in vulnerable populations. *Medical Journal of Australia*, *172*, 292–295.

McDonald, B. (2015, July 31). Humanitarian agencies need to stop failing their staff on mental health. *Guardian*. Retrieved from www.theguardian.com/global-development-professionals-network/2015/jul/31/aid-workers-casualties-mental-health

McIntosh, P. (1990). White privilege: Unpacking the invisible knapsack. *Independent School*, *49*(2), 31. Retrieved from http://people.westminstercollege.edu/faculty/jsibbett/readings/White_Privilege.pdf

Mackenzie, C., McDowell, C., & Pittaway, E. (2007). Beyond "do no harm": The challenge of constructing ethical relationships in refugee research. *Journal of Refugee Studies*, *20*(2), 299–319. doi: 10.1093/jrs/fem008

Mackintosh, K. (2000). The principles of humanitarian action in international humanitarian law. *HPG Report 5*. Retrieved from www.odi.org/uk/hpg/publications

Mailman School of Public Health. (2009). *Guide to the evaluation of psychosocial programming in emergencies*. UNICEF. Retrieved from www.cpcnetwork.org/wp-content/uploads/2014/04/UNICEF-Evaluation-of-Psychosocial-Programs-2009.pdf

Marcus, M., Yasamy, T., van Ommeren, M., Chisholm, D., & Saxena, S. (2012). Depression: A global public health concern. WHO Department of Mental Health and Substance Abuse. Retrieved from www.who.int/mental_health/management/depression/who_paper_depression_wfmh_2012.pdf

Marmot, M., Friel, S., Bell, R., Houweling, T. A., Taylor, S., & Commission on Social Determinants of Health. (2008). Closing the gap in a generation: Health equity through action on the social determinants of health. *Lancet*, *372*(9650), 1661–1669.

Mark, M. (2009, January 3). The Rwandan genocide: Role of the media, local politics and the international community. *QEssays*. Retrieved from www.qessays.com/the-rwandan-genocide-role-of-the-media-local-politics-and-the-international-community/

Marshall, A., & Batten, S. (2004). Researching across cultures: Issues of ethics and power. *Forum: Qualitative Social Research*, *5*(3), Art. 39. Retrieved from http://nbn-resolving.de/urn:nbn:de:0114-fqs0403396

Maudling, R. (2016, May 11). Aid worker security and wellbeing at the World Humanitarian Summit. Retrieved from www.linkedin.com/pulse/aid-worker-security-wellbeing-world-humanitarian-summit-maudling?trk=prof-post

Médecins Sans Frontières (MSF). (1971). Founding of MSF. Retrieved from www.doctorswithoutborders.org/founding-msf

Médecins Sans Frontières (MSF). (2011). MSF charter and principles. Document. Retrieved from www.msf.org/msf/articles/2011/03/msf-charter-and-principles.cfm.htm.

Mills, C. (2013). *Decolonizing global mental health: The psychiatrization of the majority world.* New York, NY: Routledge.

Minas, H., Wright, A., & Kakuma, R. (2014). Goals and organizational structure of the movement for global mental health. *International Journal of Mental Health Systems, 8*(31). http://doi.org/10.1186/1752-4458-8-31

Mollica, R., Cardozo, B., Osofsky, H., Raphael, B., Ager, A., & Salama, P. (2004). Mental health in complex emergencies. *Lancet, 364*(9450), 2058–2067.

Moore, C. L. (1946). Vintage season. In J. W. Campbell (Ed.), *Astounding science fiction.* New York, NY: Street & Smith.

Moran, K. (2010). Can globalization transform humanitarian aid? HuffPost Blog. Retrieved from www.huffingtonpost.com/young-professionals-in-foreign-policy/can-globalization-transfo_b_9303520.html

Movement for Global Mental Health Newsletter (MGMH). (2014, May). Interview with China Mills for the Movement for Global Mental Health newsletter. Retrieved from www.globalmentalhealth.org/newsletter_archive/newsletter-may

Murray, C. (1994). Quantifying the burden of disease: the technical basis for disability-adjusted life years. *Bulletin of the World Health Organization, 72*(3), 429–445.

National Association of Social Workers (NASW). (1999/2017). *Code of ethics of the National Association of Social Workers.* Washington, DC: NASW Press.

Ng, S. M., Chan, C. L. W., Leung, P., Chan C. H. Y., & Yau, J. K. Y. (2009). Beyond survivorship: Achieving a harmonious dynamic equilibrium using a Chinese medicine framework in health and mental health. In M. St-Onge & S. Dumont (Eds.), *Social work and global mental health: Research and practice perspectives* (pp. 63–82). New York, NY: Routledge.

Nichols, M. (2016, December 5). UN identifies 41 Burundi, Gabon troops accused of abuse in Central Africa. Reuters. Retrieved from www.reuters.com/article/us-centralafrica-un-crime-idUSKBN13U28H

Omidian, P., & Panter-Brick, C. (2015). Dignity under extreme duress: The moral and emotional landscape of local humanitarian workers in the Afghan-Pakistan border areas. In S. Abramowitz, C. Panter-Brick, & P. Piot (Eds.), *Medical humanitarianism: Ethnographies of practice* (pp. 20–41). Philadelphia, PA: University of Pennsylvania Press.

Orbinski, J. (2008) Triage: Dr. James Orbinski's Humanitarian Dilemma. Patrick Reed. Documentary. Canada. Retrieved from www.imdb.com/title/tt1158333/

Orbinski, J. (2009). *An imperfect offering: Humanitarian action in the twenty-first century.* London: Walker Books.

Orsillo, S., Roemer, L., Litz, B., Ehlich, P., & Friedman, M. (1998). Psychiatric symptomatology associated with contemporary peacekeeping. *Journal of Traumatic Stress, 11*, 609–611.

Oxfam. (2016). For human dignity. *The World Humanitarian Summit: The challenge to deliver.* Retrieved from www.oxfam.org/files/file_attachments/bp205-for-human-dignity-world-humanitarian-summit-080715-en.pdf

Oxfam America. (2017). Global refugee crisis. Oxfamamerica.org. Retrieved from www.oxfamamerica.org/take-action/save-lives/global-refugee-crisis

Oxford English Language Dictionary online. Retrieved from www.oed.com/

Patel, V. (2001). Cultural factors and international epidemiology: Depression and public health. *British Medical Bulletin, 57*(1), 33–45. doi: 10.1093/bmb/57.1.33

Patel, V. (2007). Mental health in low- and middle-income countries. *British Medical Bulletin*, 81–82(1), 81–96. https://doi.org/10.1093/bmb/ldm010

Patel, V. (2014). Global mental health: An interview with Vikram Patel. *BMC Medicine, 12*(1), 1. https://doi.org/10.1186/1741-7015-12-44

Patel, V., & Prince, M. (2010). Global mental health: A new global health field comes of age. *JAMA, 303*(19), 1976–1977. doi: 10.1001/jama.2010.616

Patrick, S. (2011, July 20). Stopping wartime sexual abuse—of men. *Atlantic*. Retrieved from www.theatlantic.com/international/archive/2011/07/stopping-wartime-sexual-abuse-of-men/242229/

Paul, C., Sanson-Fisher, R., & Carey, M. (2013). Measuring psychosocial outcomes: Is the consumer or the professional the best judge? *European Journal of Cancer Care, 22*(3), 281–288. http://doi.org/10.1111/ecc.12048

Pearce, W., & Littlejohn, S. (1997). *Moral conflict*. Thousand Oaks, CA: Sage.

Pearl, R. (2017). 3 things U.S. medicine can learn from a global humanitarian nonprofit. Forbes.com. Retrieved from www.forbes.com/sites/robertpearl/2017/08/14/can-a-humanitarian-nonprofit-help-save-american-healthcare/#3d699a706a50

Pearlman, L. A., & Saakvitne, K. W. (1995). Treating therapists with vicarious and secondary traumatic stress disorders. In C. R. Figley (Ed.), *Compassion fatigue: Coping with secondary traumatic stress disorder in those who treat the traumatized* (pp. 150–177). New York, NY: Brunner/Mazel.

Pearson, A., & Cherepanov, E. (2012). Building a disaster behavioral health response to radiological nuclear disaster. *Journal of Emergency Management, 10*(6), 413–424.

Peltz, R. J. (2003) On a wagon train to Afghanistan: Limitations on Star Trek's Prime Directive. *University of Arkansas Little Rock Law Review, 25*, 635. Available at: https://lawrepository.ualr.edu/lawreview/vol25/iss3/6

Persaud, C. (2014). European Interagency Security Forum and InterAction. NGO safety and security training project. Retrieved from www.interaction.org/sites/default/files/InterAction%20and%20EISF%20Security%20Training%20Project%202014.pdf

Pew Research Center. (2017). Numbers, facts and trends shaping your world. Pewresearch.org. Retrieved from www.pewresearch.org/fact-tank/2017

Pittaway, E., Bartolomei, L., & Hugman, R. (2010). "Stop stealing our stories": The ethics of research with vulnerable groups. *Journal of Human Rights Practice, 2*(2), 229–251.

Ponterotto, J. G., & Casas, J. M. (1991). *Handbook of ethnic/racial minority counseling research*. Springfield, IL: Charles C. Thomas.

Prince, M. (2008). Measurement validity in cross-cultural comparative research. *Epidemiologia e Psichiatria Sociale, 17*(3), 211–220.

Prince, M., Patel, V., Saxena, S., Maj, M., Maselko, J., Phillips, M. R., & Rahman, A. (2007). No health without mental health. *Lancet, 370*(9590), 859–877.

PTSD: National Center for PTSD. (n.d.). Working with trauma survivors: What workers need to know. Burnout. Retrieved from www.ptsd.va.gov/professional/provider-type/responders/working-with-trauma-survivors.asp

Reason, P., & Bradbury, H. (Eds.). (2008). *The Sage handbook of action research: Participative inquiry and practice*. Thousand Oaks, CA: Sage.

Redfield, P. (2008). Sacrifice, triage, and global humanitarianism. In M. Barnett & T. G. Weiss (Eds.), *Humanitarianism in question: Politics, power, ethics* (pp. 199–211). Ithaca, NY: Cornell University Press.

Reisch, M., & Lowe, J. I. (2008). "Of means and ends" revisited: Teaching ethical community organizing in an unethical society. *Journal of Community Practice*, *7*(1), 19–38. https://doi.org/10.1300/J125v07n01_03

Rey, J. (2014). Psychosocial support essential to Ebola response. *MSF/Doctors Without Borders*. Retrieved from www.doctorswithoutborders.org/article/psychosocial-support-essential-ebola-response

Rabionet, S. E., Santiago, E., & Zorilla C. D. (2009). A multifaceted mentoring model for minority researchers to address HIV health disparities. *American Journal of Public Health*, *99*(S1), S65–S70.

Riddell, R. (2008). *Does foreign aid really work?* Oxford: Oxford University Press.

Rieff, D. (2002). Humanitarianism in crisis: Humanitarian interventions. *Foreign Affairs*. Retrieved from www.foreignaffairs.com/articles/2002-11-01/humanitarianism-crisis

Rokeach, M. (1973). *The nature of human values*. New York, NY: The Free Press.

Rokhideh, M. (2017). Peacebuilding and psychosocial intervention: The critical need to address everyday post conflict experiences in northern Uganda. *Intervention*, *15*(3), 215–229.

Rothschild, B. (2006). *Help for the helper: Self-care strategies for managing burnout and stress*. London: W. W. Norton & Company.

Rysaback-Smith, H. (2015). History and principles of humanitarian action. *Turkish Journal of Emergency Medicine*, *15*(Suppl. 1), 5–7. http://doi.org/10.5505/1304.7361.2015.52207

Safer, D. J. (2002). Design and reporting modifications in industry-sponsored comparative psychopharmacology trials. *Journal of Nervous and Mental Diseases*, *190*, 583–592.

SanJuan, R. V. (2003). MSF position vis-à-vis Sphere Project. Position paper. Retrieved from https://web.archive.org/web/20050108170748/www.msf.fr/documents/base/2003-03-25-VilaSanJuan.pdf

Save the Children International Alliance. (1996/2010). *Promoting psychosocial well-being among children affected by armed conflict and displacement: Principles and approaches*. Geneva: International Save the Children Alliance. Retrieved from https://resourcecentre.savethechildren.net/node/3019/pdf/3019.pdf

Schmitt, E., & Shanker, T. (2005, July 26). U.S. officials retool slogan for terror war. *New York Times*. Retrieved from www.nytimes.com/2005/07/26/politics/us-officials-retool-slogan-for-terror-war.html

Schopper, D., Upshur, R., Matthys, F., Singh, J. A., Bandewar, S. S., Ahmad, A., & van Dongen, E. (2009). Research ethics review in humanitarian contexts: The experience of the independent ethics review board of Médecins Sans Frontières. *PLoS Med*, *6*(7), e1000115. doi: 10.1371/journal.pmed.1000115

Schulman, K. A., Seils, D. M., Tirnbie, J. W., Sugarman, J., Dame, L. A., Weinfurt, K. P., … Califf, R. M. (2002). A national survey of provisions in clinical-trial agreements between medical schools and industry sponsors. *New England Journal of Medicine*, *347*(17), 1335–1341.

Schwarz, N. (2000). Emotion, cognition, and decision-making. *Journal of Cognition and Emotion*, *14*(4), 433–440. http://dx.doi.org/10.1080/026999300402745

Shalala, D. E. (2000). Protecting research subjects: What must be done. *New England Journal of Medicine*, *343*, 808–810.

Sheather, J., Jobanputra, K., Schopper, D., Pringle, J., Venis, S., Wong, S., & Vincent-Smith, R. (2016). A Médecins Sans Frontières ethics framework for humanitarian innovation. *PLoS Med*, *13*(9), e1002111. https://doi.org/10.1371/journal.pmed.1002111

Shevchenko, O., & Fox, R. (2008). "Nationals" and "expatriates": Challenges of fulfilling "sans frontières" ("without borders") ideals in international humanitarian action. *Health and Human Rights, 10*(1), 109–122. doi: 10.2307/20460093

Singer, P. (1993). *How are we to live? Ethics in an age of self-interest*. Melbourne, Australia: Text Publishing Company.

Souza, A., Yasuda, S., & Cristofani, S. (2009). Mental health treatment outcomes in a humanitarian emergency: A pilot model for the integration of mental health into primary care in Habilla, Darfur. *International Journal of Mental Health Systems, 3*(1), 17.

Sphere Project. (1997). *Humanitarian charter and minimum standards in humanitarian response*. Retrieved from www.sphereproject.org/

Sphere Project. (2004). *The Sphere Project training on minimum standards in disaster response*. UK: Oxfam.

Sphere Project. (2011). *Humanitarian chapter and minimum standards in disaster response*. Geneva: The Sphere Project.

Sphere Handbook. (2014). Essential health services. *Humanitarian charter and minimum standards in humanitarian response*. Retrieved from www.spherehandbook.org/en/essential-health-services-mental-health-standard-1-mental-health/

Stamm, B. H. (Ed.). (1995). *Secondary traumatic stress: Self-care issues for clinicians, researchers, and educators*. Lutherville, MA Sidran Press.

Stevens, M. J., & Gielen, U. P. (Eds.). (2007). *Toward a global psychology: Theory, research, intervention, and pedagogy*. Mahwah, NJ: Lawrence Erlbaum Associates.

Stoddard, A., Harmer, A., & Czwarno, M. (2017) *Aid worker security report 2017. Behind the attacks: A look at the perpetrators of violence against aid workers*. Humanitarian Outcomes. USAID. www.humanitarianoutcomes.org; www.aidworkersecurity.org

Storey, A. (1997). Non-neutral humanitarianism: NGOs and the Rwanda crisis. *Development in Practice, 7*(4), 384–394. Retrieved from www.jstor.org/stable/4029004

Storr, W. (2011, July 17). The rape of men: The darkest secret of war. *Guardian*. Retrieved from www.theguardian.com/society/2011/jul/17/the-rape-of-men

Strugatsky, A., & Strugatsky, B. (2005). *Monday starts on Saturday: Fantastic story, 1965*. (A. Bromfield, Trans.). London: Seagull. (Original work published 1965)

Strugatsky, A., & Strugatsky, B. (2014). *Hard to be a god*. (O. Bormashenko, Trans.). Chicago, IL: Chicago Review Press. (Original work published in 1965)

Substance Abuse and Mental Health Services Administration (SAMHSA). (2004). *National consensus statement on mental health recovery*. Retrieved from www.samhsa.gov/recovery

Substance Abuse and Mental Health Services Administration (SAMHSA). (2014). *SAMHSA's concept of trauma and guidance for a trauma-informed approach*. HHS Publication No. (SMA) 14-4884. Rockville, MD: Substance Abuse and Mental Health Services Administration.

Summerfield, D. (1999). A critique of seven assumptions behind psychological trauma programs in war-affected areas. *Social Science and Medicine, 48*, 1449–1462.

Summerfield, D. (2002). Effects of war: Moral knowledge, revenge, reconciliation, and medicalized concepts of "recovery." *BMJ, 325*(7372), 1105–1107. Retrieved from www.ncbi.nlm.nih.gov/pmc/articles/PMC1124587/

Summerfield, D. (2004). Cross-cultural perspectives on the medicalization of human suffering. In G. M. Rosen (Ed.), *Post-traumatic stress disorder: Issues and controversies* (pp. 233–245). Chichester, UK: John Wiley & Sons. doi: 10.1002/9780470713570.ch12

Summerfield, D. (2012). Afterword: Against "global mental health." *Transcultural Psychiatry, 49*(3–4), 519–530. doi: 10.1177/1363461512454701

Summerfield, D. (2013) "Global mental health" is an oxymoron and medical imperialism. *BMJ, 346*(f3509). doi: 10.1136/bmj.f3509

Styron, W. (1979). *Sophie's choice.* New York, NY: Random House.

Tan, Y. S. & von Schreeb, J. (2015). Humanitarian assistance and accountability: What are we really talking about? *Prehospital and Disaster Medicine, 30*(3), 264–270.

Taylor, J. E., Filipski, M. J., Alloush, M., Gupta, A., Valdes, R. I., & Gonzalez-Estrada, E. (2016). Economic impact of refugees. *Proceedings of the National Academy of Science of the United States of America, 113*(27), 7449–7453. doi: 10.1073/pnas.1604566113

Tol, W. A., Stavrou, V., Greene, M. C., Mergenthaler, C., Garcia-Moreno, C., & van Ommeren, M. (2013). Mental health and psychosocial support interventions for survivors of sexual and gender-based violence during armed conflict: A systematic review. *World Psychiatry, 12*(2), 179–180. Retrieved from www.ncbi.nlm.nih.gov/pmc/articles/PMC3683274/

United Nations (UN). (2015). *Safety and security of humanitarian personnel and protection of United Nations personnel* (Resolution A/RES/70/104). Retrieved from www.un.org/en/ga/search/view_doc.asp?symbol=A%2FRES%2F70%2F104

United Nations Children's Fund (UNICEF). (2016). *New fund launches to address global education crisis.* Retrieved from www.unicef.org/media/media_91132.html

United Nations Chronicle. (2004). "Nothing about us without us": Recognizing the rights of people with disabilities. Retrieved from https://web.archive.org/web/20070614173650/www.un.org:80/Pubs/chronicle/2004/issue4/0404p10.html

United Nations Climate Change (UNCC) (2011, May 27). *Workstream III: Operational modalities transitional committee first technical workshop internal draft.* Retrieved from https://unfccc.int/files/cancun_agreements/green_climate_fund/application/pdf/tc_tsuws_ws3.pdf

United Nations General Assembly (UNGA). (1948). Universal declaration of human rights (3rd session, resolution 217). Palais de Chaillot, Paris, France. Retrieved from www.un.org/en/universal-declaration-human-rights

United Nations General Assembly (UN/IASC). (1992). *The Inter-Agency Standing Committee (IASC)* (resolution 46/182 and resolution 48/57). Retrieved from www.un.org/Docs/journal/asp/ws.asp?m=A/RES/46/182

United Nations General Assembly (UN/OCHA). (1991). *Strengthening of the coordination of humanitarian emergency assistance of the United Nations* (session 46, resolution 182, A/RES/46/182).

United Nations High Commission for Refugees (UNHCR). (1997). *Social and economic impact of large refugee populations on host developing countries* (UNHCR Standing Committee EC/47/SC/CRP.7, 6th meeting). Retrieved from www.unhcr.org/en-us/excom/standcom/3ae68d0e10/social-economic-impact-large-refugee-populations-host-developing-countries.html

United Nation High Commission for Refugees (UNHCR). (n.d.). Data. Retrieved from www.unhcr.org

Walker, P., Hein, K., Russ, K., Bertleff, G., & Caspers, D. (2010). A blueprint for professionalizing humanitarian assistance. *Health Affairs, 29*(12), 2223–2230. doi: 10.1377/hlthaff.2010.1023

Wall, I. (2016, March 21). "We are demanding change": The Somali woman taking on international NGOs. *Guardian.* Retrieved from www.theguardian.com/global-development-professionals-network/2016/mar/21/degan-ali-somali-woman-taking-on-the-humanitarian-system

Warner, G. (2017, August 28). Attempts to address rape in Congo produced unintended consequences. NPR Podcast. Retrieved from www.npr.org/2017/08/28/546668883/attempts-to-address-rape-in-congo-produced-unintended-consequences

Watters, E. (2010a) *Crazy like us: The globalization of the American psyche*. New York, NY: Free Press.

Watters, E. (2010b, January 8). The Americanization of mental illness. *New York Times Magazine*. Retrieved from www.nytimes.com/2010/01/10/magazine/10psyche-t. html?mcubz=1

Wessells, M. G. (2009). Do no harm: Toward contextually appropriate psychosocial support in international emergencies. *American Psychologist*, *64*(8), 842. doi: http://dx.doi.org/10.1037/0003-066X.64.8.842

Williams, M. B. (2010) Ethics for traumatologists. Workshop handouts. Trauma Recovery Education and Counseling Center. Warrenton, VA.

Williams, M. B. (2012). Ethics. In C. R. Figley (Ed.), *Encyclopedia of trauma: An interdisciplinary guide* (pp. 233–235). Thousand Oaks, CA: Sage.

Wilson J. (2009). Towards a normative framework for public health ethics and policy. *Public Health Ethics*, *2*(2), 184–194.

Wisner, B., & Adams, J. (Eds.). (2002). *Environmental health in emergencies and disasters: A practical guide*. Geneva: WHO. Retrieved from (www.who.int/water_sanitation_health/hygiene/emergencies/em2002intro.pdf

World Health Organization (WHO). (2001) *The world health report 2001—mental health: New understanding, new hope*. Geneva: WHO Press.

World Health Organization (WHO). (2002). *Environmental health in emergencies and disasters: A practical guide*. Geneva: WHO.

World Health Organization (WHO). (2012). *Sixty-fifth world health assembly*. Retrieved from www.who.int/mediacentre/events/2012/wha65/journal/en/index4.html

World Health Organization (WHO). (2013). *Ethical issues in patient safety research: Interpreting existing guidance*. Geneva: WHO. Retrieved from http://apps.who.int/iris/bitstream/10665/85371/1/9789241505475_eng.pdf

World Health Organization (WHO). (2017). *Responding to children and adolescents who have been sexually abused*. Geneva: WHO. Retrieved from www.who.int/reproductivehealth/publications/violence/clinical-response-csa/en/

World Health Organization (WHO/mhGap). (2008). *Mental health gap action programme: Scaling up care for mental, neurological and substance use disorders (mhGAP)*. Geneva: WHO. Retrieved from www.who.int/mental_health/mhGAP/en/

World Health Organization (WHO/nhGAP). (2010). *mhGAP intervention guide for mental health, neurological and substance use disorders in non-specialized health settings*. Geneva: WHO. Retrieved from www.who.int/mental_health/mhgap

World Health Organization, War Trauma Foundation, & World Vision International (WHO/WTF/WVI). (2011). *Psychological first aid: Guide for field workers*. WHO: Geneva.

World Humanitarian Summit (WHS). (2016). *Compact for young people in humanitarian action*. Retrieved from www.un.org/youthenvoy/wp- content/uploads/2016/05/CompactforYoungPeopleinHumanitarianAction-FINAL-EDITED-VERSION.pdf

World Medical Association (WMA). (2015). *Medical ethics manual* (3rd ed.). Ferney-Voltaire Cedex, France: John R. Williams.

Yehuda, R., & McFarlane, A. C. (2009). Is PTSD a valid diagnosis: Who benefits from challenging its existence? *Psychiatric Times*, *26*(7).

Young, H. (2015, November 23). *Guardian* research suggests mental health crisis among aid workers. *Guardian*. Retrieved from www.theguardian.com/global-development-professionals-network/2015/nov/23/guardian-research-suggests-mental-health-crisis-among-aid-workers

Index

Note: **bold** page numbers denote illustrations and *italicised* page numbers denote tables.

5Rs model (Relief, Response, Recovery, Reinforcement, Retention) 4, 12–13, *12*, 49

Abaseen Foundation 129
Abramowitz, S. 74
accountability 3, 20–21, **21–2**, 30, **32**, 35–36, 37, 41, 83, 84, 85–86, 88–90, 91, 97, 143, 144, **150**, 164; to affected populations 5, 7, *33*, 36, 38, 39, 41, 85, 86, 89, 90, 92, 96, 143, 159; central role of 2–3, 5, 9, 35, 45, *109*, 141, 161, 164, 166; and professional dilemmas 7, 103, 104, 106–107, 108–110, *109*, 141, 163; to resource-providers 41, 85, 86; *see also* "nothing about us without us"
Accountability Framework methodology 89
advocacy 52, 53, 55, 60, 61, 68, **145**
Afghanistan 157–158
Ahayalimudin, N. A. 71–72
Ahmad, R. 17
Algeria 15
Allan, T. 130
Allden, K. 64
American Counseling Association 42, 47
American Red Cross 71, 72, 90
Amnesty International 41–42
Anand, S. 24
Antares Foundation 3, 129
APA (American Psychiatric Association) 15, 42, 47, 81, 141, 142
Arendt, Hannah 122
Armenia 19, 116
aspirational values 3, 6, 7, 41, 46, 47–48, *47*, 83–93, 94, 97, 101, 139, **150**, 163
ATSS (Association of Traumatic Stress Specialists) 42, 70
Atun, R. 17
Aung, K. T. 71–72
AWSD (Aid Worker Security Database) 128

Baingana, F. 17
"Barbie savior" 123, *123*

Bartolomei, L. 42–43
Batten, S. 62
Beauchamp, T. L. 44
Behnke, S. 44, 103
Benatar, S. R. 43
Bertleff, G. 34, 35
Bhutta, Z. 64
Biafran Civil War 29
biases 8, 86, 115, 118, **120**, 141, 144, **144**, 153, 163; refugees and 9, 152, 153–154; *see also* impartiality
Biller-Andorno, N. 76, 104, 108
biomedical model of mental health 1, 23, 25, 121
Blagescu, M. 35
Bond, T. C. 11
Bosnia 16, 19
Bowie, N. E. 44
Braak, J. 70, 115
Brewer, M. B. 118
Bubenzer, F. 13, 17
Burma 146
burnout 8, 130, **131**, 132–135, **134**, 138, **145**, 162, 168; causes 6, 8, 58, 116, 132, 133, **134**; prevention and reversal 3, 131, 135, *135*, **136**, 138, 162, 163–164, 165

Cambodia 15
Candilis, P. J. 83–84, 94
capacity building 1, 6–7, 12, **13**, 26, 36, 51, 74, 77, 85, 87, **151**, 164, 165
Caplan, G. & Caplan, R. 121
Carey, M. 52
Carter Center 19, 56
Casas, J. M. 61
Caspers, D. 34, 35
CBPR (community-based psychological recovery) model **13**, 54, 56–57, 76, 99
Chechnya 56
Cherepanov, E. 6, 10, 16, 18–19, 42, 51–52, 53, 54, 55, 66, 76, 94, 116, 130, 133, 135–136, 153, 162
Chernobyl 56, 99
children as research subjects 6, 66–68
Chisholm, D. 126
Chiumento, A. 42–43, 62
Chomsky, Noam 27
civil society 34, 36
Clarinval, C. 76, 104, 108
Clark, J. 121
codes of ethics 2, 6, 42, 44, **44**, 45, 46, *46*, 47, *47*, 48, 70, 72, 85, 97–98, 123, 139, 150, 162
Cole, Teju 117, **117**
collaboration 2, 8, 11, 19, 30, 45–46, 81, 94, 116–117, 141, 144, **148**, 163; with host country 11, **13**, 87, 96, 102; multidisciplinary 2, 11, 16, 37, 46, **78**, 100, 105–106, **148**, 161, 164; in research 70, 142; *see also* integrated approaches
"colonizatory bias" 118, **120**
complex emergencies (CEs) 4, 6, 12, **12**, 16, 27, 30, 49–59, *50*, 74, 76, 77, 140
Composite International Diagnostic Interview version 2.1, 15
Comprehensive Mental Health Action Plan 2013–2020 20
confidentiality 6, 72, **78**, 107, 158; of research 6, 63, **63**, 64, 66–67, 68, 70
Congo 30, 80, 96–97, 146
Connorton, E. 129
consistency 94, 99, 141, 167
controversies 22–26
Cooper, Janice 55
Cork, Chris 129
Côte d'Ivoire 52
countertransference 6, 8, 70–71, 115–118, **120**, 121, **134**, **149**, 152, 153, 155, 156, 163
Cristofani, S. 17–18
Crittenden, C. 66, 90, 97

Darfur 18
Darou, W. 66
data ownership in research 62, **63**, 65–66
De Jong, K. 15, 16–17
de las Casa, L. 35
De Phillis, L. 71
de Torrente, N. 27–28, 43, 90
decision-making 4, 36, 43, 44, 57, 69, 71, 77, 84, 85, 95, 111, 115, 126, 146, 163, 167–168; and accountability 35, 39, 90, 106–108, 109–110, 159; and aspirational values 7, 47–48, 91–93; and professional codes of ethics 2, 42; and values-based ethical framework 2, 8–9, 44, **44**, 45,

47–48, *47*, 139, 140–141, 143, 161; *see also* "nothing about us without us"
depression 18, 19, 23, 54, 99–100, 126, 147; among aid workers 129, **131**, 132–133, 134, **134**, 136, **137**, 153
dignity 28, 38, 39, *39*, 41, 53, 68, 69, **78**, 123
dilemmas 103–104; *see also* moral dilemmas; multidisciplinary dilemmas; professional dilemmas
disability 24, 31, 36, 113, 126, **149**, 164
disaster management 6, 30, 31, **32**, 33, 34, 37, 38, 40, 41, 42, 71–72, 94, 142, 163
disaster (trauma) tourism 8, 61, 124
discrimination 20, 96, 118, **151**, 156, 165
diversification of GMH 15, 18–20, **22**, 162
"do no harm" 95, 97–98, *98*, 101, 122, **151**
Dolgoff, R. 107
"dominant culture" bias 118, **120**, 154
DSM-III (*Diagnostic and Statistical Manual of Mental Disorders*) 4, 15, **21**
"dual loyalty" dilemma 8, 130, **131**
duty to intervene **63**, 67–68

Eaton, J. 20
Ebola outbreak, West Africa 7–8, 79, 82, 101
"Education Cannot Wait" fund 31
Edwards-Levy, A. 157
Ehlich, P. 137
emotional reasoning 111, 112, *112*, 113, 141, 163
ERBs (Ethical Review Boards) 68
Ethical Rules Screen model 107
Ethiopia 15, 29, 37, 94
"ethnocentric" bias 118, **120**, 154
Everall, R. 133, 135
Everly, G. S. 99
evidence-based practices 16, 35, 67, 77, 124
"existential despair" 8, 130, 131, **131**, **134**
"expert bias" **120**, 154
"expert privileges" 119, **120**, 155
Express Tribune 128

family tracing and reunification 54
Feeny, N. C. 67
Fellenz, Martin 90
Fendrich, M. 67
Figley, C. R. 132
Flannery, R. B. 99
focused non-specialized supports 52, *53*, 54
for-profit companies 40, 84
fragmentation 1–2, 14, 15–16, **21**, 29, 37, 75, 94, 99, 100, 104, 122, **148**, **151**, 162, 164
Freud, Anna 116
Freud, Sigmund 115
Friedman, M. 137
Frith, L. 42–43

Gaza 15
GBV (gender-based violence) 16, 19, 152
Geale, S. K. 71
"gender privileges" 119, **120**, 154
Geneva Convention 128
Global Alliance for Chronic Disease 26
globalization 1, 4–5, 14, 15, 21, 24, 25, 34, 75–76, 121, 162; *see also* neocolonialism
GMH (Global Mental Health): definition 1, 4, 10–14, *12*; history of 1–2, 4, 14–22, **21–22**, **32**, 162, 166, 167
God, playing 124–126
Goodman, R. 56
Grand Challenges project 4, **22**, 26, 66
Green, B. L. 54
The Guardian 129
Guardian Global Development Professional Network 3, 129
Guidelines on Mental Health and Psychosocial Support in Emergency Settings (MHPSS) 3, 6, 7, 10, 17, 20, **22**, 30, **32**, 52–56, 85, 94–102, *109*, **151**, 161–162, 163

Habilla 18
Haiti 15–16, 19, 35, 81, 88
HAP International (Humanitarian Accountability Partnership International) 35–36, 88–89
Harris, C. E. Jr. 83, 140
Harvey, Hurricane 71
Hein, K. 34, 35
Hemenway, D. 129
heuristics 111
Hilhorst, D. 41, 84
HIV 16–17, 18, 19, 99–100
Hodgkinson, P. 136, 137

holistic approaches 13, 21, **22**, 52, **78**, 162, 164
Holtzman, S. 51
"host country" bias **120**, 154
Hugman, R. 42–43
Hum, A. 66
human rights 5, 15, 28, **32**, 38, 41–42, 65, 81, 83, 84, 95, 96–97, **151**, 158
Humanitarian Charter 5, 37–39, *39*, *40*, 45–46
Humanitarian Coalition 49, *50*
humanitarian imperative 5, 30, 41, 43, 85, 91–92, **150**
"humanitarian impunity bubble" 8, 130, **131**
humanitarian law 28, 35, 38, 40, 143
humanitarian principles 83–93, 94, 105–106, *106*, 167; aspirational nature of 3, 6, 7, 83–93, 94, 139, 163; and codes of conduct 41–42, 44, **44**, 46, *46*, 48, **150**; history of 28–31, **32**; *see also* universal humanitarian values
humanitarianism, definition of 27–28, 33
humanity as fundamental principle 28, 29, **32**, 83
"hurry up and wait" 71

IASC (Interagency Standing Committee) 6, 10, 11, **21**, 29, 30, 52–56, *53*, 60–61, 142; *see also Guidelines on Mental Health and Psychosocial Support in Emergency Settings*
iatrogenesis 23, 63–64, 121
IFRC (International Federation of the Red Cross and Red Crescent) 29, **32**, 38, 40, 83, 85, 89, 128, 141, 142, 156, 157
Illich, I . 121
impartiality 5, 27, 28, 29, **32**, **79**, 83, 86, 96, 121, 143, **150**, 156
imperative values 46, 47, *47*, 48, 139
Inayatibt, N. 71–72
independence 28, 29, **32**, 83, 86–87, 143, **150**
industrialization of humanitarianism 5, 21, 34–35
"informational privileges" 119, 154
informed consent 120, 124, *125*; in research 6, 62, **63**, 64–65, 67, 68
innovations 43, 60, 77, **78–79**
integrated approaches 11, 16–18, **21**, 45, 54, 95, 99–100, 104, **145**, 162, 164, 165; and refugees 147, **148**, 150, **151**
integrity 2, 4–5, 6, 8, 75, 84, 85–86, 94, 106, 108, 143
InterAction 51
International Save the Children Alliance 17
intervention pyramid 52, *53*
IPV (intimate partner violence) 18
Iraq 146, 157–158
Italy 41

Jenkins, R. 17
Jenson, E. 6, 42, 71
Johnson, T. P. 67
Josephson Institute of Ethics 107
Jung, Carl 115

Kakuma, R. 20
Karadag, O. C. 77–78
Katz, C. L. 11
Katz, P. A. 117
Kerim Hakan, A. 77–78
Khan, M. N. 42–43
Kipling, Rudyard 117, 118
Kirmayer, L. J. 24
Kodner, D. L. 17
Kohlberg, L. 9, 143
Kohrt, B. A. 44, 143–144
Koplan, J. P. 11
Koppel, T. 137
Kosovo 19, 30, 56
Kouchner, Bernard 29
Kurtness, J. 66

Labott, S. M. 67
Lambert, J. 60, 63, 64
language barriers 58, 81, **149**, **150**
Last Mile-Health 19, 52, 55
Leaning, J. 64, 68
Lerner, M. J. 116
Lewis, D. 32
Liberia 19, 52, 53, 54, 55, 56, 74
Life Events and Social History Questionnaire 15
Lipsky, S. 118
Lister, G. 43

Littlejohn, S. 105
Litz, B. 137
LLMIC (low- and low middle-income countries) 20, **22**, 33–34, 64, 74, 75, 126–127, 163
Lloyd, R. M. 35, 36
Locke, P. 22–23
Loewenberg, F. M. 107
London School of Hygiene and Tropical Medicine 26

Mackenzie, C. 42
Mackintosh, K. 33–34
Mailman School of Public Health 23–24
Marcus, M. 126
Marienfeld, C. B. 44
Marshall, A. 62
Martinez, R. 83–84, 94
McDaid, D. 17
McDonald, Brendan 129
McDowell, C. 42
McIntosh, P. 119, 154
McLaughlin-Rotman Centre for Global Health 26
Mental Health General Action Plan 2013–2020 10
Merson, M. H. 11
MGMH (Movement for Global Mental Health) 20, **22**, 26
mhGAP (Mental Health Global Action Plan) 4, 13, 20, **22**, 55
MHPSS (mental health and psychosocial interventions and supports) 6, 10, 13, 60–61, 74; *see also Guidelines on Mental Health and Psychosocial Support in Emergency Settings*
Miller, D. T. 116
Miller, M. 129
Mills, China 25–26, 75, 118
Minas, H. 20
"missionary bias" 118, **120**
Mollica, R. 19
Monrovia 79
Moore, C. L. 124
moral dilemmas 9, 44, 45, 57, 58, 70, 95, 110–112, *112*, 133, **136**, 142–143, **144**, **149**, 163, 168
moral reasoning 111, 112, *112*, 113, 141, 163
morality, post-conventional 9, 143
Moran, K. 34
MSF (Médecins Sans Frontières/Doctors Without Borders) 17–18, 19, 29, 38, 43, 69, 77, **78–79**, 101, 128, 135
Mueller, Kayla 172–173, *173*
multidisciplinary dilemmas 3, 4, 7, 104–106, *106*, 141, 163, 170
multidisciplinary humanitarianism 2, 14, 16, **21**, 28, 38, **44**, 45–46, *47*, 58, 76, 95, 99–100, 141, **145**, 150
multilayered supports 95, 100–101, **151**

Nairobi 90
National Association of Social Workers 42, 47
needs-based model 6, 104, 164
neocolonialism 24, 25–26, *25*, 75–76, 118, 126
neutrality 5, 28, 29, **32**, 37, 40, 65, 83, 87, **150**, 157
Ng, S. M. 164
NGOs 28, 31, 32, 35; Code of Conduct 5, 8, 30, **32**, 37, 38, 40–42, 84, 130
Nigeria 29
NIMH (National Institute of Mental Health) 26
normative (binding) values 5, 6, 8, 42, 43–44, **44**, 45, 46, 47, *47*, 62, 71, 106, 140
"nothing about us without us" 5, 36, 88–90, 97, 159
Nurumal M. S. 71–72

OCHA (Office for the Coordination of Humanitarian Affairs) 29, **32**
Ogard, Beathe 123–124
operational guidance 2, 3, 6, 7, 46, *46*, 47–48, *47*, 84, 91, 95, 139–140, **150**, **151**, 167; *see also Guidelines on Mental Health and Psychosocial Support in Emergency Settings*
operational modality 12, **12**, **13**, 49
Orbinski, J. 106
Orsillo, S. 137

Pakistan 128–129
"Palava" tradition 57

Panter-Brick, C. 44
Papua New Guinea 19
PAR (participatory action research) standards 64
participation 95, 96, **151**
Partners in Health 19
Patel, V. 11, 23, 24, 25, 165
pathologizing paradigm of Western mental health 1, 11, 14, 23, 24–25, 63–64, 161
Patrick, S. 96
Paul, C. 52
Paulson, B. 133, 135
peace building 13, **13**, 21, **22**, 51, 77, 105, 164
Pearce, W. 105
Pearl, R. 9, 165–166
Pearlman, L. A. 132
Pedersen, D. 24
peer support 8, 111, 134–135, **136**, 137, **144**, **145**, **148**, 155, 159
Peltz, R. J. 76
Perry, M. J. 129
Persaud, C. 129
Pew Research Center 146
pharmaceutical companies 25, 26, 121, 126
Philippines 19
photographs 123–124, *123*, *125*
Pittaway, E. 42–43, 61–62, 119–120
Ponterotto, J. G. 61
post-conflict settings 6–7, 13, 72–76, *73*, 77, 122, 140, 163
post-conventional morality 9, 143
power differentials 8, **63**, 64, 67, 75, 118–119, **120**, 122, 144, 151, 152, 154
prejudices 8, 118, **120**, **144**
prescriptive values 46, 47, *47*, 48
Prince, M. 11, 25, 64
prioritizing needs 2, 3, 7, 41, 71, 75, 77, 85, 90, 96, 104
prioritizing values 2, 45, 46–48, *47*, 95, 96, 103, 105–106, 107, 108
privileges 115, **117**, 118–119, **120**, 152, 154, 158–159, 163
professional competencies 1, 2–3, 4, 5, 6, 9, 21, 35, 70, 71, 85, 140, 141–145, **144–145**, **150**
professional dilemmas 2, 3–4, 7–8, 42, 58, 106–110, 133, 141
professional reasoning 111, *112*, 113, 141, 163
professionalization 4, 15, 16, 20–21, **22**, 26, 34–35, 42, 62, 129, 143, 166
proselytizing 5, 87, **150**
psychosomatic complaints 18, 19, 54
psychotropic medications 56, 102, 121, 124, 126–127
PTSD (post-traumatic stress disorder) 4, 15, **21**, 23; among aid workers 129, 132, 133

quality control 2, 12, 19, 21, **22**, 30, 35–36, 37, 38, 62, 88–89, 106, 164

Rabionet, S. E. 65
Rahman, A. 42–43, 71–72
rational reasoning 8, 111, *112*, 113, 141, 163
Recamier, Max 29
recovery 49–52, 56–57, 73–74, 76, 81, 92, 97, 99, **149**, **151**, 164; *see also* 5Rs model
Red Cross *see* IFRC
reentry 8, 102, 134–138, **134**, **137**
referral systems 6, **13**, 54, 55, 58, **63**, 70, 72, 135, 147, 156
refugee law 35, 38, 143
refugees 9, 16, 30, 31–32, 41, 52, 53, 65, 88, 119, **145**, 146; research with 68, 69; in United States 9, 146–160
rescuer fantasy 8, 116–117, **120**, 130, **131**, **134**, 153
research, humanitarian 42–43, 60–70, **63**, 124, 142, 163, 165; on children 6, 66–68
Riddell, R. 32
RMH (refugee mental health services) 146–160, **148–149**, **150–151**
Robert S. Strauss Center for International Security and Law 50
Roemer, L. 137
Rokeach, M. 44
Rokhideh, M. 13, 74, 77, 104, 105, 122
Russ, K. 34, 35
Russia 19, 84–85
Rwanda 29, 35, 37
Rysaback-Smith, H. 28, 32–33, 83, 94

Saakvitne, K. W. 132
safety 3, 6, 8, 27–28, 30, 31, 58, 91, 118, 128–138, **131**, 139, 141, **144**, 162, 163, 165, 171; as ethical responsibility 4, 8, 45, 46, *46*, 47, *47*, 48, 95; and refugees **148**, 151, 152, 159–160; and research 62, 64, 65, 66–67, 68, 124
SAIH (Students' and Academics' International Assistance Fund) 123–124, *123*, *125*
SAMHSA (National Consensus Statement on Mental Health Recovery) 56, **148**
sampling in research **63**, 64, 65
Sanson-Fisher, R. 52
Santiago, E. 65
Save the Children 17, 141
Saxena, S. 126
Schopper, D. 68
Schuetz-Mueller, J. 11
Schwarz, N. 111
SDH (social determinants of health) 11, 17
Segall, M. 117
self-awareness 2–3, 4, 45, 95, 103–104, 135, 141, **144–145**, 163; and cognitive distortions 115, 116, 118, 153
self-care 3, 4, 6, 95, 116, 128–38, **144–145**, 155, 159, 162, 163–164, 171; as ethical requirement 4, 6, 8, 45, 46, *46*, 47, *47*, 48, 70, 71
"sense of stage" 8, 122–124, *123*, 159
Seven Hills International 19
sexual exploitation and abuse 67, 75, 80, 90, 96–97, 100–101, 120; by aid workers 30, **32**, 88, **150**
Sheather, J. 43, 77
Sierra Leone 19
Singer, P. 65
social media 123–124, *123*, *125*
"socioeconomic privileges" 119, **120**, 154
Somalia 146, 157
Sophie's Choice 110
Souza, A. 18
Sphere Project 5, 29, 30, 33, *33*, 37–39, *39*, *40*, 45, 57, 85, 104–105
Spreeuwenberg, C. 17
Stamm, B. H. 132
Star Trek 75–76
stereotypes 90, 115, 118, **120**, 123, 124, *125*, 152, 154
Stewart, M. 136, 137
stigma 14, 18, 20, 24, 54, 55, 56, 57, 109, **145**, **149**, **151**, 152
Stobbaerts, E. 43, 90
Storey, A. 29
Strugatsky, Arkady and Boris 76, 98
Styron, William 110
Sudan 17–18, 19
Summerfield, D. 23, 25, 75, 121
survivor guilt 8, 112, 116, 117–118, **120**, 131, **134**, **137**, **149**
SWWS (Support With Working Solution) 129
Syria 19, 146

Tajikistan 19
Tan, Y. S. 89
Tankink, M. 13, 17
TB (tuberculosis) 16–17, 18, 19
temoignage (testimony) 79, 80, **145**
TFT (Thought Field Therapy) 81
Thacker, S. C. 43
Thailand 119, 120
training **13**, 143–144, 163, 165, 167–171
transparency 83, 91, 92, 102, 104, 106, **148**
trauma 1, 15, 18, 19, 24, 25, 30, 51, 54–56, 57, **151**, 156; and aid workers 70, 98, 111, 112, 115, 129, 130, 132–133, 136, **137**, **145**, 153, 159, 163; and ethics 6, 42, 70–71, 115–116, 152, 162; and refugees 9, 147, **148**, 152, 153; secondary trauma 133; *see also* PTSD
trauma (disaster) tourism 8, 61, 124
Tsai, A. C. 44
tsunami (Asia, 2004) 35

Uganda 74, 77, 104, 122
Ukraine 56
UN (United Nations) 20, **21**, 28, 29, 30, 37, 61, 88, 96, 146
UNHCR (High Commission for Refugees) 31–32, 53
UNICEF 17, 141
Universal Declaration of Human Rights 28
universal humanitarian values 2, 9, 14, 28, 31, 34, 83, 84, 105, 143, 150, 161, 163

validity of research 6, 61, 63–64, **63**, 66, 69
values-based framework for GMH ethics 2–3, 5, 8–9, 14, 43–48, **44**, *46*, *47*, 108, 139–145, 161, 162–163; and professional codes of ethics 44, **44**, 45, 46, *46*, 47, *47*, 48; in refugee mental health 150–152, **150**
van Ommeren, M. 126
victim blaming 116, **120**, **134**
von Schreeb, J. 89
vulnerability 1, 6, 9, 24, 28, 38, 41, 49, *50*, 51, 57, 61, 66, 75, **78–79**, 115, **149**; of aid workers 132, **136**; not exploiting 5, 83, 87–88, **150**

Wainberg, M. L. 44
Walker, P. 34, 35, 143
"war of paradigms" 4–5, 23
War Trauma Foundation 13
Warner, G. 80
Watters, E. 25, 75
Wellcome Trust 26
Wessells, M. G. 64
West Africa 30, 56–57, 79, 82
White guilt 117, **120**
"White privilege" 119, **120**, 154
White savior complex 117, **117**
WHO (World Health Organization) 11, 13, 19–20, **22**, 24, 27, 50, 67, 68, 126, 128
WHS (World Humanitarian Summit, 2016) 30–31, 34, 51, 129
Williams, M. B. 6, 42, 70–71, 115, 116
Wilson, J. 104
WMA (World Medical Association) 98
World Vision International 13, 19
Wright, A. 20

Yasamy, T. 126
Yasuda, S. 18

Zorilla, C. D. 65